MRCOG Part 2

Comprehensive Preparation Manual

OSCE

A. RAHIM KASSID HALOOB,
MB, ChB, FRCOG, FFFP
Consultant Obstetrician and Gynaecologist
Basildon University Hospital, UK
Honorary Professor of Obstetrics and Gynaecology
Basrah University, Iraq

ALI IZZET NAKASH
MBChB, MRCOG, DRCOG
Speciality doctor in Obstetrics and Gynaecology
North Middlesex University Hospital, UK

Volume 3 OSCE

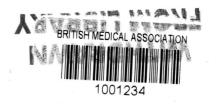

ISBN: 1496036832
ISBN 13: 9781496036834

Library of Congress Control Number: 2014903789
CreateSpace Independent Publishing Platform
North Charleston, South Carolina

Comprehensive Preparation Manual

Volume Three, OSCE

Contents

Further Readings xv

Acknowledgments xvi

Section 1 1

General 1

OSCE Section of Final MRCOG Examination 1

How to Pass and Score High 2

1-History and Communication Stations 2

2-Examination Stations 3

3-Skills Station and Communications 3

4-Data Interpretation 4

5-Gallery Station 5

6-Design Audit Project 5

Contents

HOW TO...undertake a clinical audit 6

Process for Undertaking a Clinical Audit 9

Monitor implementation of action plan 11

7) Design Local Guideline to Be Used in Your Department 12

8) Write Patient Information Leaflet 12

9) Handover and Labour Ward Prioritization 13

The board display should show the following: 13

Section 1 34

Communications and Consent 34

Consent 34

To Aid the Consent 35

Obtaining Consent... 35

Establishing Capacity to Make Decision... 36

Best Interests Principle.. 36

Types of Consent... 37

Case 1 37

Case 2 37

Section 2 40

Gynaecology.. 40

History OSCE Stations 40

Candidate Instructions.. 40

Part 1 41

Part 2 41

Examiner Instructions 41

Marking Sheath 42

Reference 44

Gynaecology OSCE Station 45

Recurrent Miscarriage (RM) 45

Candidate Instructions.. 45

Examiner Instructions 45

Marking Sheet 46

References 48

Gynaecology OSCE Station 50

Pelvic Endometriosis/Abdominal Pain 50

Contents

Candidate Instructions 50

Part 1 50

Part 2 51

Part 3 51

Examiner Instructions 51

Marking Sheath 52

OSCE Station 56

Heavy Menstrual Bleeding (HMB) 56

Candidate Instructions 56

The Letter 56

Role-Player Information 57

Examiner Instructions 58

Marking Sheet 58

Reference 64

Gynaecology OSCE Station 65

Abnormal Cervical Smear 65

Candidate Instructions 65

Role-Player Information..65

Examination Instruction...66

Marking Sheet...67

Menstrual Dysfunction..70

Gynaecology OSCE Station...70

Candidate Instructions..70

Examiner Instructions...70

Marking Sheet...71

Reference..73

Subfertility Station..74

Gynaecology OSCE Station...74

Candidate Instructions..74

Part 1...74

Part 2...74

Examiner Instructions...75

OSCE Station..78

Fertility 2...78

Contents

Candidate Instruction..78

Examiner's Instruction 79

Marking Sheet 80

Ovulation disorders..83

Gynaecology OSCE Station 87

Uterine Fibroids 87

Candidate Instructions 87

Examiner Instructions 88

Marking Sheet 88

OSCE Station 93

Urogynaecology station...93

Candidate Instructions...93

Referral Letter..93

Part 1 93

Part 2 94

Examiner Instruction...96

Marking Sheet 97

Obstetric and Gynaecological History 99

Physical Examination.. 101

Neurophysiology 101

OSCE Station 104

Amenorrhoea.. 104

Candidate Instruction.. 104

GP Letter 104

Part 1 105

Part 2 105

Examiner Instructions 105

Marking Sheet 107

Follicle Depletion 110

Section 3 116

Obstetrics 116

OSCE Stations 116

Candidate Instructions... 116

Marking Sheet 118

Contents

Station 2 121

Risk Management 121

Candidate Instructions 121

Letter 121

Examiner Instructions 122

Marking Sheet 122

OSCE Station 124

Respiratory Disease 124

Candidate Instruction 124

Examiner Instructions 124

Marking Sheet 125

ORAL CORTICOSTEROIDS 129

References 131

Monochorionic Twin Gestation 132

OSCE station 132

Candidate Instructions 132

Examiner Instructions 132

Marking Sheet 133

References 137

Sickle Cell Disease (SCD) 138

OSCE Station 138

Candidate Instructions 138

Examiner Instructions 138

Marking Sheet 139

Thromboembolism (VTE) 144

OSCE Station 144

Candidate Instructions 144

Examiner Instructions 144

Marking Sheet 145

OSCE Station 149

Preterm Labour 149

Candidate Instructions 149

Role-player Instructions 149

Examiner's Instructions 150

Contents

Marking Sheet 151

OSCE Station 155

No Foetal Movements... 155

Candidate Information 155

Role-Player Information.. 155

Marking Sheet 158

Obstetrics OSCE Station 162

Postnatal Collapse.. 162

Candidate Instruction.. 162

Second part 163

Third Part.. 164

Fourth Part 164

Examiner's Notes... 165

Marking Sheet 166

Amniotic Fluid Embolism 167

Obstetrics Preparatory OSCE Station 169

Medicolegal Case... 169

Candidate Instruction... 169

Obstetric OSCE Station... 175

Medicolegal Case... 175

Examiner Instruction... 175

Marking Sheet 178

Obstetrics OSCE Station.. 182

Mental Diseases.. 182

Candidate Instructions... 182

Examiner Instructions.. 182

Marking Sheet 183

Obstetrics OSCE Station.. 187

Ovarian Cyst during Pregnancy.. 187

Candidate Instruction... 187

Part 1 187

Part 2 187

Examiner Instruction... 188

Marking Sheet 189

Contents

References 192

Obstetrics OSCE Station 193

Gestational Diabetes 193

Candidate Instruction... 193

Examiner Instructions 193

Marking Sheet 195

References 202

FURTHER READINGS

1-Green Top RCOG Guidelines: www.rcog.org.uk/guidelines

2-NICE Guidelines in Obstetrics and Gynaecology: www.nice. org.uk

3-GMC Guidance and Instructions/Good Medical Practice (2013): www.gmc-uk.org/guidance

4-Society of Gastrointestinal & Endoscopic Surgeons (SAGES): www.sages.org/publications/guidelines

5-British Fertility Society Guidelines: www.britishfertilitysociety. org.uk

6-British Society of Gynaecological Endoscopy: www.bsge.org.uk

ACKNOWLEDGMENTS

We would like to thank Miss Nora Haloob MRCS, ENT (Glasg) for her contribution to the sections Breaking Bad News and Communications OSCE Stations and her advice in the setting of other OSCE stations.

SECTION 1

GENERAL

OSCE Section of Final MRCOG Examination

Candidates who pass the written examination must sit the oral examination immediately following. The written mark does not contribute towards the oral score. The Part 2 MRCOG oral examination consists of twelve stations. Ten of these stations will have an examiner present, and two will be preparatory stations for the following one. Each station is fifteen minutes long, with one minute of that being initial reading time.

The format of questions may be as follows:

1-You may be asked to describe an operation in detail, which may include preoperative and postoperative discussions.

2-Your communication skills will be assessed by your interaction with a role-player depicting a particular scenario.

3-Your history-taking skills may be assessed.

4-You may be presented with a clinical problem and asked to explain it to a role-player.

5-You may be faced with a number of clinical problems and have to prioritise what needs to be done and by whom.

6-You may be asked to describe, demonstrate, or assemble some surgical equipment or teach skills using it.

7-You may be asked to design an audit protocol.

8-You may be asked to appraise critically an information leaflet.

Each of the ten active stations carries equal marks.

How to Pass and Score High

The OSCE section of the final MRCOG examination is three hours long: the morning session is from 09.00 until noon, and the afternoon session from 13.30 to 16.30. This is a very taxing time and requires good mind and body preparation. A good rest period before the examination with a small meal will do your body and mind good. Timekeeping is controlled electronically with a bell at the beginning and end of the fifteen-minute station and at the end of the first minute. Stay calm.

1- History and Communication Stations

These stations are manned by one examiner and one actor (role-player). The examiner has no active role, and his interaction is minimal. The actor is your patient, and you have to blind your mind to this fact and take her role as real and factual, behave as you would with your patient in your daily clinical practice. The interaction with the patient at the beginning is a general approach, moving to specific issues.

The opener must be a direct question to the patient to explain to you her compliant and how this is affecting her daily work, living, and relations. There might be a hidden intention in this scenario you have to discover from minor hints in the history of the patient.

Example: a twenty-three-year-old Somalian emigrant was admitted via the accident and emergency A&E department with lower abdominal pain and feeling unwell; during history you might discover that the station centred on female genital mutilation.

2- Examination Stations

No role-play or patient is involved; you may be asked to talk about an instrument and conduct your examination on a manikin. As in a normal clinical set-up, be confident, fluent, and go to the basics: adopting the normal modified process of an inspection, palpation, and auscultation approach.

In each OSCE station, always introduce yourself and gain consent and cooperation of the patient by saying *Good morning, I am Dr. David Martin. I would like to ask you few questions; do you have an objection?* If your patient gave a history as per a scenario of pain, ask if she is in pain at the moment.

3- Skills Station and Communications

The GMC document titled "Good Medical Practice" identifies communication as a key area, and you are expected to work in partnership with patients and to listen and respond to their concerns. You should be able to give patients information as per their requests regarding what they want or need in a way that they can understand.

Good team-working and communication are essential for effective handover; shift-work patterns that lead to less continuity of care have an impact on patient safety.

You may be asked to teach your junior doctor how to perform certain tasks or skills or to demonstrate, assemble, or talk about some surgical instrument. You may be asked to relay certain clinical scenario in an emergency set-up, which requires input from your senior. This depends on your presentation, which impacts the final clinical decision.

You have to name the instrument or the object given to you to inspect; for example, "This is a silicone ventouse cup." You then have to move on, describing the components of the instrument and how they function and for what purpose they are used: for example, "The plastic cup fits on the foetal head at the specific location on the head. This cup is attached to pressure plunger to create a negative pressure inside the cup to produce a chignon. The pressure must be built fast to reach the maximum allowed but must stay in the green zone of the plunger. Once the optimum pressure is reached, the pulling must be directed downward and forward to achieve head flexion to bring the shortest diameter of the head down." You have to follow the RCOG guideline for operative vaginal delivery. Then you have to talk about the requirement before applying the instrument and the limitation of its use, and talk about the complications that can affect the mother and the baby. You need to talk about the preparation prior to application and what precaution you have to take to minimise complications and make the silicone ventouse cup an effective instrument.

4- Data Interpretation

This station would cover any laboratory data and sometime statistical ones. For this station you need to name the test, date of the test, and name and hospital number of the patient. In certain circumstances you can identify in which clinical scenario these tests have been requested. You then have to analyse the data and give your conclusion and put a management plan in place.

5- Gallery Station

A pictures gallery could be for instruments, pathological specimen, clinical lesions, or histology slides. In this station, candidates might encounter any of these in a preparation station followed by discussion or a role-play station. If the test or the information is not enough to cover all aspects of the clinical scenario, you have to be prepared to instigate a further set of investigations. A pathological photo could be challenging, but knowing the tissue type is important before trying to identify the abnormality in the picture.

6- Design Audit Project

Here you should follow the audit cycle: you need to choose the audit subject, find out the current national or local guideline and best medical practice or good clinical control trial or meta-analysis by looking into the Cochran database.

You have to identify the issue or issues you are auditing against the guideline and design pro forma for data collection and where to get the data from: that is, patient records, EMR (electronic medical records), the information department, or laboratory data. You have to decide the number of records to be reviewed to make a good conclusion and recommendations. You have to obtain the agreement from the audit lead and get support from the audit department and local statistician.

Once you complete the data collection, you need help with data analysis and to decide on the conclusion and recommendations and final presentation.

Every audit with recommendations should lead to change in the way you practice; therefore, you need to decide about re-auditing after a period of time.

The audit topic is very important one; it is something you need to know in details when you are practicing in the United Kingdom. For more details about audit related issues, see below:

HOW TO...undertake a clinical audit

Choosing your topic for clinical audit

- Select a topic. Choose something that you know about, that would benefit from being audited and a topic where there are **standards** to audit against. For help see guidance leaflets on **HOW TO... tell what clinical audit is** and **HOW TO...choose and prioritise clinical audit projects.**

- Discuss your project aim with your colleagues and your audit supervisor (for doctors in training) or line manager and get their support.

Registering your clinical audit

- Obtain a *Clinical Audit Registration Form* from the clinical effectiveness unit (CEU) in the education centre or the clinical audit office in CTC, and complete Part 1.

- Provide information on who will be participating in the clinical audit, remembering to think *multidisciplinary* and *clinical team* mind-set. Consider the clinical audit aim, rationale, referenced standards, and what changes in patient care may result from the clinical audit.

- The proposal form needs to be signed by your audit supervisor (for doctors in training) or your line manager and by the clinical audit lead for your directorate/specialty.

- Staff in the CEU will talk through the clinical audit with you, reviewing aims and helping with objectives, checking standards and references, and considering methodology and sampling, data analysis, and implications for change in practice. Be realistic; make sure that what you are planning to do is achievable within the time you have to do the clinical audit.

- CEU staff will provide you with information and advice on the audit and will be able to obtain patients' notes if required, but please ensure that you give plenty of notice.

Stages of a clinical audit

- Agree on aims, objectives, method, and sample.

- Identify the sample. This does not need to be large; CEU staff can help with this.

- Design a data collection form, keeping it simple and clear. Collect only data that relates to your objectives and with a minimum of information that identifies the patient.

- Keep data secure, and maintain confidentiality.

- For data collection be consistent, objective, and accurate, data should be validated and quality-checked by someone independent to ensure it is correct.

- For data analysis, keep it simple, using percentages and averages and checking that your figures add up.

- Write a report: this should include rationale, aim, objectives, standards, references, method, sample, findings, discussion, conclusions, and recommendations for change.

- Prepare a presentation: keep it clear and concise and easy to understand; summarise key points and use charts for reporting results.

What to do when you have presented your clinical audit

- Complete Part 2 of the *Clinical Audit Registration Form* obtainable from CEU. Record your findings, proposed changes, and details of your action plan to implement the changes.

- Ensure your action plan is implemented. You may need support from your audit supervisor (for doctors in training) or your line manager and colleagues.

- Once any changes have been implemented, this topic can be reaudited to confirm an improvement in patient care, closing the clinical audit cycle.

- Congratulate yourself, and look forward to seeing your project published in the *Clinical Audit Annual Report*.

Process for Undertaking a Clinical Audit

A SIMPLE AUDIT CYCLE

Have we made
things better?

What are we trying
to achieve?

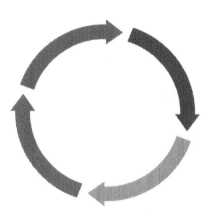

Are we doing something
to make things better?

Are we
achieving it?

Why are we not achieving it?

| Select an audit topic |

| Discuss audit with Manager/Supervisor/Audit Lead

Obtain audit registration form from CEU or intranet |

| Complete Part 1 of clinical audit registration form
– to be countersigned by Line Manager or
Audit Supervisor and Clinical Audit Lead |

| Return part completed registration form to CEU

Audit facilitation in CEU |

| Agree any recommendations for change in
practice

Agree an action plan

Complete Part 2 of registration form – to be
countersigned by line manager/ consultant |

| Monitor implementation of action plan |

| Data collection

Data analysis, Prepare Report, present findings

Prepare report

Present findings |

| When changes are in place re-audit to confirm
better practice and complete the audit cycle |

Agree any recommendations for change in practice

Agree an action plan

Complete Part 2 of registration form – to be countersigned by line manager/ consultant

Re-audit when changes are in place to confirm better practice and complete audit cycle

Monitor implementation of action plan

When changes are in place, reaudit to confirm better practice and complete the audit cycle.

7) Design Local Guideline to Be Used in Your Department

Often you are asked to design a guideline for clinical management. The local management guideline is often based on national guidelines (RCOG, NICE, GMC, British Societies guidelines) or good medical practice (clinical control trial, meta-analysis, and Cochrane reviews). Management plan should be multidisciplinary, shared, and ratified by all involved.

8) Write Patient Information Leaflet

A patient information leaflet is an integral part of good medical practice. It has to be written in simple and plain language, putting in mind that the patient has no medical knowledge and has no knowledge of any medical jargon. Basic information about the procedure should be discussed and why the patient should have the procedure and if there are any alternatives.

The patient should be told what to expect before, during, and after the procedure and the expected length of stay in hospital.

Consider possible major and minor complications that may happen during the course of treatment and the way you are going to deal with them. The patient should be informed about the length of stay in hospital, length of time needed to be off work, and the degree of limitation of activities after the procedure.

9) Handover and Labour Ward Prioritization

Handover has been the cornerstone of changes in our practice and the major change that has lead to improvement in the patient's care.

Handover in obstetrics is based on the labour ward board. This is a large board, often located in the office of the labour ward, where midwives and doctors often interact and discuss patients' care and plans of action.

The board display should show the following:

- The room number

- The name of the patient, age, and parity

- The names of her consultant and midwife in charge of her care while on the labour ward

- Her latest brief observations re time of the last vaginal examination, dilation, station of the presenting part, status of the liquor, major medical and obstetric complications, and her analgesia status. (See figure 1).

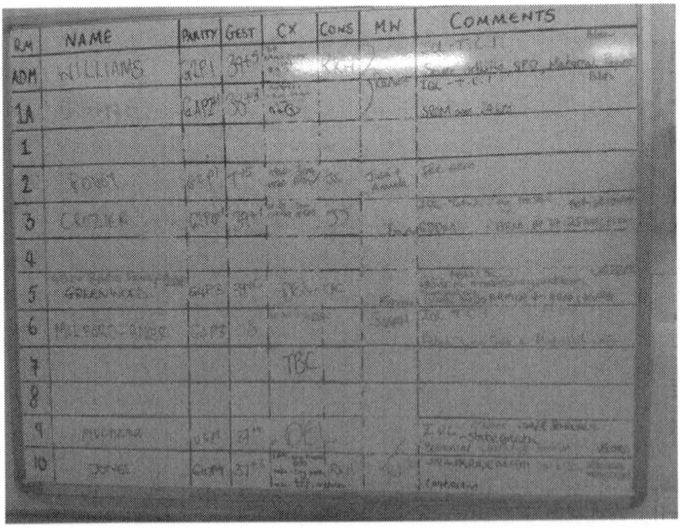

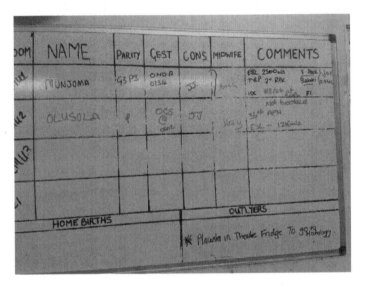

Figure 1: Labour Ward Board, updated continuously by midwives

Figure 2: Supplementary board for HDU, CMU,
with information about home births and outliers

- In modern obstetrics practice in the United Kingdom, we added to the board two items (figures 2 and 3).

1-Labour Ward High Dependency Unit (HDU)/Close Monitoring Unit (CMU). This unit is housing patients in need of intensive monitoring after or before any intervention. This could be postpartum haemorrhage more than 1 000 ml, unstable blood pressure (BP), a diabetic patient with unstable blood-sugar control, severe preeclampsia, or any patient after caesarean section (CS) in need of close monitoring for a few hours before transferring her to care in the postnatal ward.

The Modified Early Obstetric Warning Scoring observation chart (MEOWS) has been used for this purpose for the last few years and proved to be effective in early identification of abnormal signs that might call for intervention. The MEOWS chart also help with early transfer of patients from CMU or HDU to the normal maternity ward for normal observations (see figure 3). It is colour-coded, and the score is calculated from one to six and over. Level zero is an indication of normality and patient's readiness for transfer.

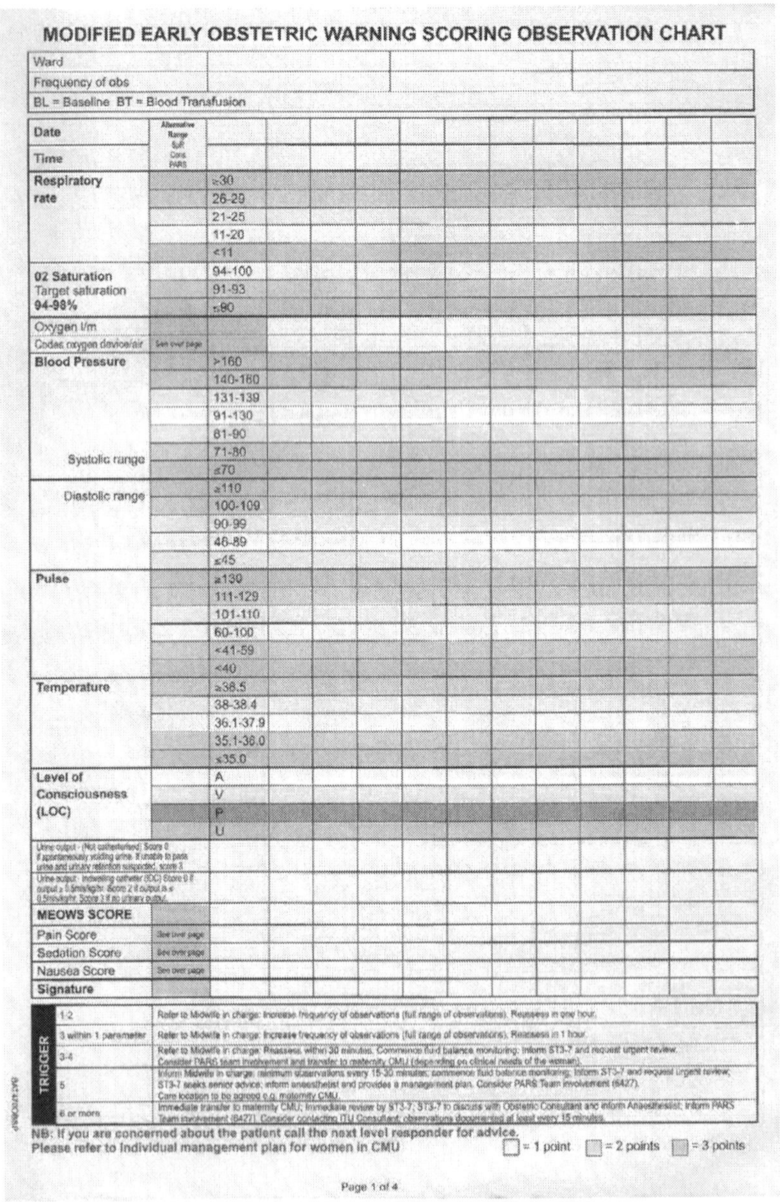

MODIFIED EARLY OBSTETRIC WARNING SCORING OBSERVATION CHART

Ward															
Frequency of obs															
BL = Baseline BT = Blood Transfusion															

	Alternative Range Suff Cons PARS														
Date															
Time															
Respiratory rate	≥30														
	26-29														
	21-25														
	11-20														
	<11														
02 Saturation Target saturation **94-98%**	94-100														
	91-93														
	≤90														
Oxygen l/m															
Codes: oxygen device/air See over page															
Blood Pressure	>160														
	140-160														
	131-139														
	91-130														
	81-90														
Systolic range	71-80														
	≤70														
Diastolic range	≥110														
	100-109														
	90-99														
	46-89														
	≤45														
Pulse	≥130														
	111-129														
	101-110														
	60-100														
	<41-59														
	<40														
Temperature	≥38.5														
	38-38.4														
	36.1-37.9														
	35.1-36.0														
	≤35.0														
Level of Consciousness (LOC)	A														
	V														
	P														
	U														
Urine output - (Not catheterised) Score 0 if spontaneously voiding urine. If unable to pass urine and urinary retention suspected, score 3. Urine output - indwelling catheter (IDC) Score 0 if output ≥ 0.5ml/kg/hr. Score 2 if output is < 0.5ml/kg/hr. Score 3 if no urinary output.															
MEOWS SCORE															
Pain Score	See over page														
Sedation Score	See over page														
Nausea Score	See over page														
Signature															

TRIGGER		
1-2	Refer to Midwife in charge; Increase frequency of observations (full range of observations). Reassess in one hour.
3 within 1 parameter	Refer to Midwife in charge; Increase frequency of observations (full range of observations). Reassess in 1 hour.
3-4	Refer to Midwife in charge; Reassess within 30 minutes. Commence fluid balance monitoring; Inform ST3-7 and request urgent review. Consider PARS team involvement and transfer to maternity CMU (depending on clinical needs of the woman).
5	Inform Midwife in charge; minimum observations every 15-30 minutes; commence fluid balance monitoring; Inform ST3-7 and request urgent review; ST3-7 seeks senior advice; inform anaesthetist and provides a management plan. Consider PARS Team involvement (6427). Care location to be agreed e.g. maternity CMU.
6 or more	Immediate transfer to maternity CMU; Immediate review by ST3-7; ST3-7 to discuss with Obstetric Consultant and inform Anaesthetist; Inform PARS Team involvement (6427). Consider contacting ITU Consultant; observations documented at least every 15 minutes.

NB: If you are concerned about the patient call the next level responder for advice.
Please refer to Individual management plan for women in CMU   ☐ = 1 point ☐ = 2 points ☐ = 3 points

Figure 3: MEOWS Chart

	3	2	1	0	1	2	3
Resp rate	≤11			11-20	21-25	26-29	≥30
O Sat %	≤90	91-93		94-100		>	≤
Systolic BP	<71	71-80	81-90	91-130	131-139	140-180	>180
Diastolic BP	≥110	100-109	90-99	47-89	≤ 45		
Pulse	<40	41-59		60-100	101-110	111-129	≥130
LOC				Alert	Voice	Pain only	Unconscious
Temperature	≤35	35.1-36		36.1-37.9	37-38.4	> 38.5	
Urine output	NIL output			≥0.5mls/kg/hr		<0.5mls/kg/hr	

Codes for recording oxygen delivery on observation chart

A   Air (not including oxygen. or weaning or on PRN oxygen

N   Nasal cannulae

SM   Simple mask

V24   Venturi 24%

V28   Venturi 28%

V31   Venturi 31%

V35   Venturi 35%

V40   Venturi 40%

V60   Venturi 60%

H28   Humidified oxygen at 28% ("Respiflow" or similar device) (also H35, H40, H60 for humidified oxygen at 35%. 40%, 60%)

RM   Reservoir mask

TM   Tracheostomy mask

CP   Patient on CPAP

NIV   Patient on NIV system

Other device (specify which):

AVPU = Alert; Voice, Pain, Unresponsive

Pain Scores	Sedation Scores	Nausea Scores
0 - No pain at rest, no pain on movement	0 - Alert	0 - None
1 - No pain at rest, mild pain on movement	1 - Occasionally drowsy easy to rouse	1 - Occasional nausea (no vomit)
2 - Mild intermittent pain at rest, moderate pain on movement	2 - Often drowsy. easy to rouse	2 - Vomit
3 - Continuous pain at rest, severe pain on movement	3 - Difficult to rouse	
	S - Normal sleep, easy to rouse	

Figure 4: Interpretation of the Information on the MEOWS Chart and Calculation of MEOWS Score/upside down

2-Patients who were admitted to the main hospital intensive care unit or critical care unit (ITU or CCU) for intensive observations such as eclampsia and severe HELLP syndrome (hemolysis, elevated liver enzymes, low platelet count) or patients with medical complications. Up-to-date information should be obtained from the ITU regularly to update the staff on the labour ward about the patient's progress while on the ITU and in order to organise time for her to return to the labour ward. Communication is paramount with the anaesthetic team and other professional groups involved in her management.

The handover time is normally at 08:00, 13:00, and 17:00, and often there is another handover at 20:00. In the consultant-led unit, the staff present in the handover are the consultant on call for labour ward, registrar, and senior house officer (SHO; ST1-7), accompanied by the lead midwife in charge of the labour ward for the shift—in addition, an anaesthetic consultant and registrar and occasionally paediatric consultant or registrar, especially for the 08:00 handover.

During the handover the consultant must go through the board and put the following in action:

- Prioritization according to clinical presentation and urgency of intervention and ability of the consultant's individual team members to deal with these priorities as per seniority.

- Plan the management of individual patient and write and sign the plan in the patient's record.

- Take immediate action to deal with any urgent situation.

- Inform the anaesthetic team about this plan.

- Inform the special care baby unit (SCBU) about any possible admission as a result of urgent intervention.

1-Cardiotocogram (CTG) Interpretation

Patients admitted to a high-risk labour ward should be monitored electronically. **High risks include the following:**

<u>Maternal medical illness</u>

Gestational diabetes

Hypertension

Asthma

<u>Obstetric complications</u>

Multiple gestation

Postdate gestation

Previous caesarean section

Intrauterine growth restriction

Premature rupture of the membranes

Congenital malformations

Oxytocin induction/augmentation of labour

Preeclampsia

<u>Other risk factors</u>

No prenatal care

Smoking

Drug abuse

Staff should have proper training in CTG interpretation and recognition of suspicious or abnormal trace, have regular updates, and be properly certified.

* Electronic foetal monitoring was first introduced in order to identify baby hypoxia in order to avoid cerebral palsy; however, only 10 to 20 percent of occurrences of cerebral palsy can be traced back to an insult during intrapartum care. Occurs in approximately two per one thousand births.

* Approximately 80–90 percent of cases are due to antenatal events (most commonly intrauterine infection).

To interpret a CTG, you need a structured method of assessing its various characteristics.

The most popular structure can be remembered using the acronym DR C BRAVADO:

DR –   Define Risk
C –   Contractions

BRa –   Baseline Rate

V –   Variability
A –   Accelerations
D –   Decelerations
O –   Overall impression

Individual contractions are seen as peaks on the part of the CTG monitoring uterine activity.

You should assess contractions for the following:

- **Duration**—*How long do the contractions last?*

- **Intensity**—*How strong are the contractions? (assessed using palpation)*

Baseline Rate
=====

The baseline rate is the average heart rate of the foetus in a ten-minute window. Look at the CTG and assess what the average heart rate has been over the last ten minutes. Ignore any accelerations or decelerations. A normal foetal heart rate is between 110 and 160 bpm.

Foetal Tachycardia

Foetal tachycardia is defined as a baseline heart rate greater than 160 bpm.

It can be caused by the following:

- Foetal hypoxia

- Chorioamnionitis—*if maternal fever also present*

- Hyperthyroidism

- Foetal or maternal anaemia

- Foetal tachyarrhythmia

Foetal Bradycardia

Foetal bradycardia is defined as a baseline heart rate less than 110 bpm.

Mild bradycardia of between 100 and 110 bpm is common in the following situations:

- Postdate gestation

- Occiput posterior or transverse presentations

Severe prolonged bradycardia (less than 80 bpm for more than three minutes) indicates severe hypoxia.

Causes of prolonged severe bradycardia are as follows:

- Prolonged cord compression

- Cord prolapse

- Epidural and spinal anaesthesia

- Maternal seizures

- Rapid foetal descent

If the cause cannot be identified and corrected, immediate delivery is recommended.

Variability

Baseline variability refers to the variation of foetal heart rate from one beat to the next. Variability occurs as a result of the interaction between the nervous system, chemoreceptors, baroreceptors, and cardiac responsiveness.

Therefore it is a good indicator of how healthy the foetus is at that moment in time. This is because a healthy foetus will be constantly adapting its heart rate to respond to changes in its environment. Normal variability is between 10 and 25 bpm. To calculate variability you look at how much the peaks and troughs of the heart rate deviate from the baseline rate *(in bpm)*.

Variability can be categorised as follows:

- Reassuring—more than or equal to 5 bpm

- Nonreassuring—less than 5 bpm for between forty and ninety minutes

- Abnormal—less than 5 bpm for more than ninety minutes

Reduced variability can be caused by the following:

- Foetus sleeping—*this should last no longer than forty minutes—most common cause*

- Foetal acidosis (due to hypoxia)—*more likely if late decelerations also present*

- Foetal tachycardia

- Drugs—*opiates, benzodiazepines, methyldopa, magnesium sulphate*

- Prematurity—*variability is reduced at earlier gestation (less than twenty-eight weeks)*

- Congenital heart abnormalities

Accelerations

Accelerations are an abrupt increase in baseline heart rate of more than 15 bpm for more than fifteen seconds. The presence of accelerations is reassuring. Antenatally there should be at least two accelerations every fifteen minutes. Accelerations occurring alongside uterine contractions are a sign of a healthy foetus. However, the absence of accelerations with an otherwise normal CTG is of uncertain significance.

Deceleration

Decelerations are an abrupt decrease in baseline heart rate of more than 15 bpm for more than fifteen seconds. There are a number of different types of decelerations, each with varying significance.

Early deceleration

Early decelerations start when uterine contraction begins and recover when uterine contraction stops. This is due to increased foetal intracranial pressure causing increased vagal tone. It therefore quickly resolves once the uterine contraction ends and intracranial pressure reduces. This type of deceleration is therefore considered to be physiological and not pathological.

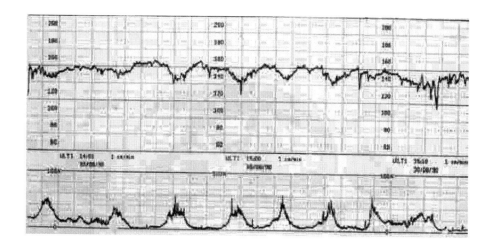

Variable deceleration

These decelerations are variable in their duration and may not have any relationship to uterine contractions. They are most often seen during labour and in patients with reduced amniotic fluid volume.

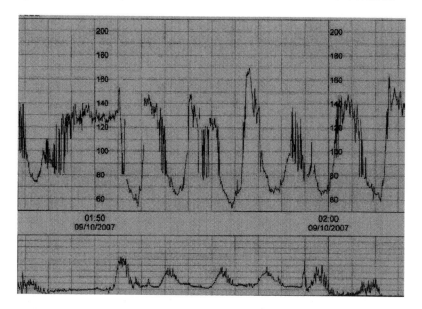

Figure 5: Variable Decelerations

Variable decelerations are usually caused by umbilical cord compression:

- The umbilical vein is often occluded first, causing an acceleration in response.

- Then the umbilical artery is occluded, causing a subsequent rapid deceleration.

- When pressure on the cord is reduced, another acceleration occurs, and then the baseline rate returns.

- Accelerations before and after a variable deceleration are known as the "shoulders of deceleration."

- Their presence indicates the foetus is not yet hypoxic and is adapting to the reduced blood flow.

Variable decelerations can sometimes resolve if the mother changes position.

The presence of persistent variable decelerations indicates the need for close monitoring.

Variable decelerations without the shoulders are more worrying, as it suggests the foetus is hypoxic.

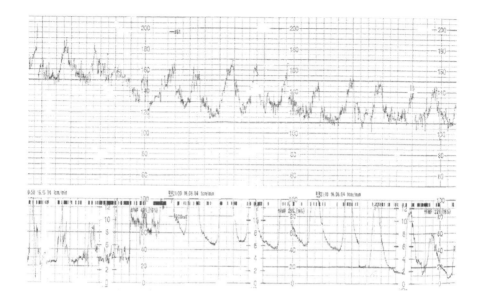

Figure 6: Another Form of Variable Decelerations.
Notice the high baseline.

Late Deceleration

Late decelerations begin at the peak of uterine contraction and recover after the contraction ends.

This type of deceleration indicates there is insufficient blood flow through the uterus and placenta.

As a result blood flow to the foetus is significantly reduced, causing foetal hypoxia and acidosis.

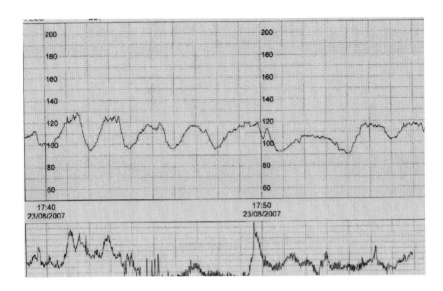

Figure 7: Flat Trace Due to Foetal Hypoxia

Reduced utero-placental blood flow can be caused by the following:

• Maternal hypotension

• Preeclampsia

• Uterine hyperstimulation

The presence of late decelerations is taken seriously, and foetal blood sampling for pH is indicated.

If foetal blood pH is acidotic, it indicates significant foetal hypoxia, and the need for emergency delivery may be by caesarean section.

Prolonged Deceleration

Prolonged deceleration is a deceleration that lasts more than two minutes.

If it lasts between two and three minutes, it is classed as nonreasurring.

If it lasts longer than three minutes, it is immediately classed as abnormal.

Action must be taken quickly—for example, foetal blood sampling / emergency CS.

Sinusoidal Pattern

This type of pattern is rare; however, if present, it is very serious.

It is associated with high rates of foetal morbidity and mortality.

It is described as follows:

- A smooth, regular, wavelike pattern

- Frequency of around two to five cycles a minute

- Stable baseline rate around 120–160 bpm

- No beat-to-beat variability

A sinusoidal pattern indicates

- severe foetal hypoxia,

- severe foetal anaemia, and

- foetal/maternal haemorrhage.

Immediate caesarean section is indicated for this kind of pattern. Outcome is usually poor.

Overall Impression

Once you have assessed all aspects of the CTG, you need to give your overall impression.

The overall impression can be described as

- reassuring,

- suspicious, or

- pathological.

The overall impression is determined by how many of the CTG features were either reassuring, nonreassuring, or abnormal. The NICE guideline below demonstrates how to decide which category a CTG falls into.

<u>The CTG monitoring must contain the following information about the patient:</u>

1) Date and time of the commencement of the CTG monitoring.

2) Name, date of birth, and hospital number.

3) During the course of monitoring, the carer must indicate any procedure done, such as epidural, vaginal examinations, top-up of the epidural, or any other intervention during labour or abnormal findings.

Table 1: NICE Classification and CTG Interpretation

* NICE CLASSIFICATION

Feature	Baseline (bpm)	Variability (bpm)	Decelerations	Accelerations
Reassuring Features	110–160	≥ 5	None	Present
Non-reassuring Features	100–109 161–180	< 5 for 40–90 minutes	Typical variable decelerations with over 50% of contractions, occurring for over 90 minutes Single prolonged deceleration for up to 3 minutes	The absence of accelerations with otherwise normal trace is of uncertain significance
Abnormal Features	< 100 > 180 Sinusoidal pattern ≥ 10 minutes	< 5 for 90 minutes	Either atypical variable decelerations with over 50% of contractions or late decelerations, both for over 30 minutes Single prolonged deceleration for more than 3 minutes	

STAN Monitoring

The modern obstetric care has acquired another tool with which we can study the ST changes in the PQRST of the foetal heart. This is a computer-driven tool in which the computer should study the normal heart trace for at least twenty minutes to decide on the future heart-trace abnormalities; therefore, it is not suitable for an already pathological trace. With a suspicious trace bordering on pathological, the status of the foetal pH and base access should be known before commencement of the STAN monitoring. The following table has been adopted by the NICE guideline to make interpretation of the recording of STAN machine:

Table 2: STAN Foetal Heart Interpretation

STAN CTG classification

CTG classification	Baseline heart frequency	Variability Reactivity	Decelerations
Normal CTG	• 110-150bpm (110 - 160 NICE)	• 5-25bpm • Accelerations	(No decelerations NICE) • Early decelerations • Uncomplicated variable decelerations with a duration of less than 60 seconds and loss of less than 60 beats
Intermediary CTG (non reassuring/suspicious NICE)	• 100-110bpm • 150-170bpm (160 - 180 NICE) • Short bradycardia episode (up to 3 minutes)	• Greater than 25bpm without accelerations • Less than 5 bpm for more than 40 minutes (40 - 90 mins NICE)	(Early/variable decelerations NICE) • Uncomplicated variable decelerations with a duration of less than 60 seconds and loss of more than 60 beats
	• A combination of several intermediary observations will result in an abnormal CTG		
Abnormal CTG (Pathological NICE)	(Less than 100bpm NICE) • 150-170bpm and reduced variability • More than 170bpm (180 NICE) • Persistent bradycardia (More than 3 minutes NICE)	• Less than 5bpm for more than 60 minutes (90 minutes NICE) • Sinusoidal pattern (Sinusoidal for more than 10 minutes NICE)	(Atypical variable NICE) • Complicated variable decelerations with a duration of more than 60 seconds • Repeated late decelerations
Preterminal CTG	• Total lack of variability and reactivity with or without decelerations or bradycardia		

The annotations in italics represent the additional guidance from NICE. The STAN system falls within the parameters of NICE.

SECTION 1

Communications and Consent

Consent

A successful doctor and patient relationship depends on trust, respect of patient's autonomy, and effective and strong communication.

Patients have the right to be fully informed about their condition and the treatment offered. They essentially should know about the following:

- Diagnosis and prognosis

- Uncertainties about the diagnosis

- Options of treatment / management

- Purpose of proposed investigation and treatment

- Likely benefits and probabilities of success

- How and when condition will be monitored

- Doctor overall responsibility

- Involvement of doctors in training and students

- Availability of second opinion

- The possibility of any additional problems and the need for consent to deal with these problems

To Aid the Consent

The patient needs up-to-date written material and visual and other aids.

Language of communication must be adequate for the doctor and the patient to understand each other.

There should be sufficient time to digest the information and contact information with available support groups and nursing and other health-care members.

Obtaining Consent

This must be done by a qualified doctor with sufficient training and knowledge to deal with all aspect of treatments offered.

Delegation must be to suitably trained and qualified staff who will act in accordance with GMC guidance.

Balanced view should be delivered with honesty.

Every adult has the capacity to make decision; fluctuating capacity calls for review of competence.

In mentally incapacitated patients, management needed should be delivered in the best interest of the patient. A court order is needed for nontherapeutic or controversial treatment.

Establishing Capacity to Make Decision

- Children age sixteen or older make decisions; however, for patients under sixteen, establishing capacity depends on the level of understanding. If a competent child refuses treatment, parents/court authorises treatment in the best interest of the child.

- For patients detained by police, for immigration services, and for mental-health legislation, the best interest issues must be applied.

- In emergencies, treatment can be given; however, this is limited to only life-saving or preventing significant deterioration in patient health.

Best Interests Principle

- Options clinically indicated.

- Patients previously expressed preferences and made advance statements.

- Patient background, culture, religious, or employment considerations.

- Views of third party.

- Option should least restrict patient future choices.

- Doubt legal advice.

Types of Consent

- Verbal consent.

- Implied consent; be careful.

- Written consent, close to time of treatment.

- Consent for screening.

- Consent to research—this needs written consent; results are not predicted, and consent requires understanding the research project.

- Multimedia images—imaging for teaching, education, and publications.

Case 1

The patient is forty-five years old, and this is an egg donation pregnancy; she has a history of pulmonary embolism at eighteen years old, when the patient was on oral contraceptive pill.

Case 2

The patient is a twenty-six-year-old woman in her second pregnancy. Her first baby delivered at 32+5.

The placenta showed thrombosis and, being small, no family history of thrombosis.

Currently on aspirin and Clexan.

12- Breaking Bad News and Role-Playing

1. Impact of environment on consultation

- Furniture set up—appropriate distance, not across a table; ensure nonhostile environment to build rapport

- Ensure no distractions—no bleep/mobile phones.

2-Introduction

- Introduce by name, shake hands (if patient accepts), show patient to his or her seat.

- Ask the patient if there is a relative or friend to be with them during the consultation.

- Explain the objectives of the consultation, giving a brief overview of how it will run.

3- Opening statement—check understanding.

4. Give bad news:

- Do not delay the issue.

- Give time for patient to take it in.

- Offer empathy.

5. Explore patient's distress.

6. Continue to show empathy throughout consultation.

7. Offer contact details, supplement information (leaflets, website, support groups).

8. End consultation by summarizing the forward plan.

Remember: body language, nonjudgmental attitude, empathy but not sympathy, reassurance but not false promises.

SECTION 2

GYNAECOLOGY

History OSCE Stations

Stations with history have been dominating the OSCE examination of Part 2 MRCOG examination since its introduction. Each scenario has a short introduction, which has to be read and understood; formalise initial structured answer for one minute before entering the station. The scenario is still available to be reviewed inside the station. There might be secondary and tertiary scenarios during station discussion. There is no requirement to examine the patient, but you have to prepare a solid plan for management.

Candidate Instructions

You are a year three registrar at the antenatal clinic. Mrs. K. Timson came to her first visit with you at sixteen weeks' gestation. She is thirty-two years old and a full-time medical secretary.

She is para one: she delivered vaginally and had uncomplicated antenatal period in her previous pregnancy.

This time she has been having pains all over her body, since she stopped her medication, which was prescribed by her rheumatologist. She told you that she is still on her injection for antiphospholipid syndrome.

Part 1

1-Take full obstetrics history.

2- Take full medical history.

Part 2

She told you that she was doing well during her first pregnancy without medications, unlike the current pregnancy, and that she cannot carry on without medication for her pain.

1- Put an action plan for her medical care.

2- Agree a plan with this patient with regard to the antenatal care.

3- What is the post delivery and future plan?

Examiner Instructions

Mrs. Timson is thirty-two years old and has a known case of rheumatoid arthritis under Professor Chacravarti and has been doing well while under methotrexate, which she stopped when she found that she was pregnant.

Her rheumatoid factor was high, and they found that she has high level of antiphospholipid antibodies and was advised to be on Clexan 40 mg during pregnancy.

She was referred for physiotherapy, which was of little benefit.

She was telling you that she has been feeling progressively more pain in her joints and has been taking more time off.

Marking Sheath

1- History of her condition prior to the
last pregnancy and after.   0 1 2

2- How she managed her last labour and delivery.   0 1 2

3- Write to her previous hospital about first pregnancy.   0 1 2

4- Write to her doctor about her rheumatoid arthritis.   0 1 2

5- Multidisciplinary approach.   0 1 2 3

6- Plan her antenatal care and medication
required to control her pain.   0 1 2

7- Pain clinic   012

8- Get the advice of Prof. Chacravarti regarding
the current condition.   0 1 2

9- Social services.   0 1

10- Liaise with employer to adjust her work pattern.   0 1

Discussion

This is a case of rheumatoid arthritis (RA) with active disease during pregnancy in addition to positive APA. Her current condition is affecting the following:

Her ability to function at home and work

Progress of her pregnancy

Expected complication

This complex case can be managed only by a multidisciplinary team.

RA affects nearly one in ten thousand people in the general population and affects more women than men (3:1). The peak prevalence is age thirty to fifty years. It is characterised by fatigue, joint pain and deformity, and extra-articular manifestations, including pleurisy, pericarditis, subcutaneous nodules, and pulmonary fibrosis.

At least 49 percent (De man et al. 2008) of cases improved during pregnancy, and the peak improvement occurs in the second or third trimester; some reported disappearance of rheumatic nodules during pregnancy. This improvement is with variable degree, and there is no clinical prediction to indicate the improvement in RA during pregnancy. This improvement is still with no clear mechanism, as the correlation with the level of cortisone is poor, and oestrogen and progesterone do not benefit RA. However, maternal immune response to paternal HLA antigens may have a role in pregnancy-induced remission.

Nearly three quarters of those improved will relapse in postnatal period.

Non steroidal anti-inflammatory agents (NSAIDs) should be avoided, and glucocorticoids should be considered for those who did not improve during pregnancy.

Some progressive diseases during pregnancy may necessitate the use of medications to modify the disease. Hydroxychloroquine has some foetal toxicity, but very small, and sulfasalazine has no adverse foetal effect. D-penecillamine is contraindicated in pregnancy because of impaired foetal connective tissue formation, and gold salt may be safe to use in pregnancy.

Methotrexate is contraindicated during the first trimester and should be stopped in the prepregnancy period.

Reference

1. de Man, Y. A.; Dolhain, R. J.; van de Geijn, F. E.; Willemsen, S. P.; Hazes, J. M.

Disease activity of rheumatoid arthritis during pregnancy: results from a nationwide prospective study. *Arthritis Rheum.* 2008; 59(9):1241–8.

Gynaecology OSCE Station

Recurrent Miscarriage (RM)

Candidate Instructions

You are sitting in gynaecology outpatient. Mrs. L. is your first patient on the list. She is thirty-two years old, generally fit, and healthy. Her mood seems very low. The GP tell you in his letter that she been trying for a family for five years, but every time she gets pregnant, it ends up in a miscarriage either first or second trimester. This happened for four consecutive times.

1) What is she suffering from? And how you going to assess her?

2) How you going to investigate her?

3) What are the treatment options?

Examiner Instructions

Mrs. L. is thirty-two years old, para zero plus four, and had four miscarriages: the first at fourteen weeks, which was lost spontaneously, and the second one at twelve weeks, for which the patient needed surgical evacuation for retained products. The last two miscarriages happened at ten weeks, which happened spontaneously. In the last two pregnancies, she was prescribed folic acid and aspirin to be taken from early pregnancy.

The gynaecology history of notice is the history of one termination of pregnancy at the age of sixteen, which was done medically; however, she needed subsequent evacuation for retained products.

The family history includes early father death at the age of forty-four from possible pulmonary embolism, but that was never confirmed. Mother suffers from SLE for many years, for which she was put on immunosuppressant recently in view of the severity.

She smokes ten cigarettes/day, and she is working hard to reduce it and stop it eventually. She was referred by her GP recently to the smoking cessation programme, and she already attended a few sessions. She might go for the nicotine patches soon.

Marking Sheet

1) What is she suffering from? And how you going to assess her?

Recurrent miscarriage	012
Detailed history of miscarriages	012
Past personal medical history	012
Past family history	012
Social and drug history	012

2) How you going to investigate her?

Antiphospholipid antibodies	012
Karyotyping	012
Pelvic ultrasound	012
Thrombophilias screen	012

Laparoscopy/hysteroscopy if indicated 012

3) What are the treatment options?

Treat the cause 012

Low dose aspirin plus heparin 012

Referral to clinical geneticist if needed 012

Cervical cerclage if needed 012

Tender loving care 01

Discussion

One of the most important aspects of care in these couples is the need for constant reassurance and alleviation of anxiety, because there is considerable psychological pressure on the part of the patient and the doctor. Make sure that if surgical evacuation is needed, specimen should be sent for foetal karyotype, and a full autopsy examination is needed for midtrimester loss. During any operative intervention, it is important to document any suspected uterine abnormalities.

Routine investigations of recurrent miscarriage is an important baseline investigation before embarking on much advance further investigations such as antibodies check and thrombophilia screening. Further investigation must be directed by positive history findings and examination. This should include anatomical disorders of the uterus and cervix, which may lead to RM and premature labour.

Family history is often forgotten in history taken but may have the key cause of RM, such as in this case, with a strong family history of SLE and thrombophilia disorders. Endocrine causes are hard to confirm, but some data are suggestive of some protective effect of progesterone in idiopathic RM.

Routine testing of woman with no history suggestive of diabetes for diabetes mellitus is unnecessary. Empirical therapy is unjustifiable.

There must be an agreed-upon and clearly documented plan for management and monitoring in a subsequent pregnancy. An early first trimester transvaginal scan is valuable, to confirm viability early in pregnancy, and regular scans during second trimester to exclude any abnormalities, such as incompetent cervical, so provide additional reassurance. Prophylactic dexamethasone may be considered from twenty-four weeks' gestation.

During the third trimester, serial scans are advisable for woman at risk of premature labour and perinatal death.

References

1. Stirrat, G. M. Recurrent miscarriage. *Lancet* 1990; 336:673–5.

2. Wyatt, P. R.; Owolabi, T.; Meier, C.; and Huang, T. Age-specific risk of fetal loss observed in a second trimester serum screening population. *Am J Obstet Gynecol* 2005; 192:240–6.

3. NyboAnderson, A. M.; Wohlfahrt, J.; Christens, P.; Olsen, J.; and Melbye, M. Maternal age and foetal loss: population based register linkage study. *BMJ* 2000; 320:1708–12.

4. Regan, L.; Braude, P. R.; and Trembath, P. L. Influence of past reproductive performance on risk of spontaneous abortion. *BMJ* 1989; 299:541–5.

5. de la Rochebrochard, E.; and Thonneau, P. Paternal age and maternal age are risk factors for miscarriage; results of a multicentre European study. *Hum Reprod* 2002; 17:1649–56.

6. Clifford, K.; Rai, R.; and Regan, L. Future pregnancy outcome in unexplained recurrent first trimester miscarriage. *Hum Reprod* 1997; 12:387–9.

7. Lindbohm, M.L.; Sallmén, M.; and Taskinen, H. Effects of exposure to environmental tobacco smoke on reproductive health. *Scand J Work Environ Health* 2002; 28 Suppl 2:84–96.

8. Rasch, V. Cigarette, alcohol, and caffeine consumption: risk factors for spontaneous abortion. *Acta Obstet Gynecol Scand* 2003; 82:182–8.

9. Peck, J.D.; Leviton, A.; and Cowan, L. D. A review of the epidemiologic evidence concerning the reproductive health effects of caffeine consumption: a 2000–2009 update. *Food Chem Toxicol* 2010; 48:2549–76.

Gynaecology OSCE Station

Pelvic Endometriosis/Abdominal Pain

Candidate Instructions

You are a registrar in the gynaecology clinic.

Mrs. J. Lawson, thirty-eight years old, came to you complaining of lower abdominal pain and irregular periods for the last eight months.

Her periods have been painful, erratic, and heavy, preceded by two to three days of feeling unwell, hot flushes, irritability and agitation, and shouting at her only child.

She has had the same features in 2010, prior to her infertility investigations, and had to have a laparoscopy. She delivered her child two years ago normally.

Part 1

1- Take a full history.

2- Take relevant information about the operation she had in the past.

3- List your plan of action.

Part 2

She told you that she was trying to conceive for two years, and, after removal of her endometriomas by laparoscopy, she had to have IVF treatment.

1- Take specific history of her fertility.

2- Enquire about the outcome of IVF.

Part 3

She mentions to you that she is fed up and wants permanent treatment of her pain, because it is interfering with her job, relation, and daily routines, as she has been in pain for eight months and wants a hysterectomy but is reluctant, because she is still thinking about having another baby.

In 2012–2013 she had three failed IVFs and was told that her egg quality was poor.

1- Advise on what to do and what are her options.

2- Tell your plan to fulfil her desire for another baby.

Examiner Instructions

This patient has severe pelvic endometriosis, and infertility and laparoscopy revealed stage four endometriosis. Surgical procedure improved her fertility, leading to induction of ovulation for four months and intrauterine insemination (IUI) for three months. Then she was treated with IVF when she got pregnant after first attempt. She delivered normally at full term.

She came back after one year and wants to get pregnant with another IVF treatment.

Her hormonal profile showed slightly elevated follicle-stimulating hormone (FSH) at 11.5 u/L, and her AMH level was 6.5 pmol/L.

She had three attempts of IVF but no pregnancy.

She was advised on egg donation.

This time her main problems are her period and pain interfering with her job, relation, and daily routines. She wants to have definitive treatment: total abdominal hysterectomy (TAH) and bilateral salpingo-oophorectomy (BSO). However, she is still thinking of how can she get pregnant and at the same time cannot carry on with the pain and periods problems.

Marking Sheath

Full and comprehensive menstrual history

Frequency

Duration

Character of the periods

Pain before and during   0 1 2 3

Enquire about the operation she had in 2010

Laparoscopic finding

What has been said about fertility

Why she has to have IVF

Discuss what is your management plan   0 1 2 3 4

Fertility history

Any male factor

Initial hormonal profile in 2010

Any treatment prior to IVF   0 1 2 3

Discuss the outcome of IVF

Number of retrieved eggs

Number of fertilised eggs

Number of embryos transfer   0 1 2 3

Options available

TAH + BSO + hormone replacement therapy (HRT)

Implication of long term HRT

BSO and preservation of uterus and egg donation   0 1 2 3 4 5 6

Discussion

Endometriosis is a chronic inflammatory and sometimes debilitating disease with pelvic pain affecting the life and relationship of the woman. The disease is sustained by aberrant expression of several proinflammatory cytokines. Epidemiological studies suggest that women with certain forms of endometriosis may have an increased risk of preterm birth and small for gestational age. The possible mechanisms are of altered endometrial function and prostaglandin (PG) levels. However, women with endometriosis are more likely to have difficulties conceiving and more likely to receive assisted reproduction technology (ART).

The inflammatory response to pelvic endometriosis causes adhesions that further increase the morbidity of the disease; this will trigger period pain, dyspareunia, dyschezia, and alteration of bowel habits. Progressive pelvic disease might result in severe genitourinary damage affecting bladder and ureteric function and blockage due to anatomical distortion. Careful history-taking, including family history, and careful assessment of the woman's symptoms to include regularity and heaviness of her periods, dysmenorrhea, pelvic pain, dyspareunia, bowel and urinary symptoms, upper GI symptoms such as nausea and vomiting and bloating, and inguinal pain have to be obtained on direct questionings. Pelvic and abdominal examination as well as utilising imaging investigations will help in planning of management.

Radical surgery does not guarantee no recurrence of the disease, and loss of fertility might be one of its drastic outcomes; alternative treatment should be offered, especially when there is a desire for future pregnancy.

A heavy and irregular period is one of the presentations and often does not implicate the uterus. Failure of this patient to respond to conservative surgical intervention might push the gynaecologist to think of bilateral salpingo-oophorectomy and preservation of uterus and future fertility, knowing that she will need egg donation anyway. We always have to remember that for women who wish to preserve their fertility, the rate of recurrence of pain is 44 percent with surgical management and 53 percent with medical management.

In this case there are several issues:

1- This patient has had three failed IVFs with poor follicular growth. Her anti-Müllerian (AMH) is low indicating low ovarian reserve. The next step in her infertility management will be egg donation.

2- Her current and acute presentation is her pelvic pain and dysmenorrhoea. This has its impact on her daily routine, and this can affect her sexual relation. She demanded definitive treatment.

3- Medical treatment in this case has little or no role apart from temporary pain relief. Surgical treatments could be as follows:

    A- Laparoscopic approach with ablation of pelvic endometriosis followed by GnRh down regulation and pursuit of egg donation.

    B- Laparoscopy with an option of bilateral salpingo-oophorectomy for severe endometriosis and followed by egg donation.

OSCE Station

Heavy Menstrual Bleeding (HMB)

Candidate Instructions

The patient you about to see has been referred to your outpatient clinic by her general practitioner. A copy of the letter is given below.

Read the letter; obtain a relevant history from the patient. You should discuss any relevant investigations and treatments that you feel are indicated.

The examiner will provide you with the results of the pelvic examination when requested.

The Letter

Dear Gynaecologist,

I would be grateful if you could see Ann Flood; age 41. She has been having increasingly heavy period over the last year and has failed to respond to medical treatment.

Yours sincerely,

Dr. M. Smith, MRCGP

You will be awarded marks for your ability to take a history and explain investigations and treatment to the patient.

Role-Player Information

You are forty-one years old and have two children, both born by caesarean sections for foetal distress. Your periods have been getting heavier over the past year, since you were sterilised.

You are happily married and work as a care assistant.

Your periods are regular, coming every thirty days, and last up to eight days, with clots and occasional soiling of your clothes. Staining of bed linen is more frequent. For sanitary protection you need to wear maxi pads most of the time. However, periods are not very painful.

Your social activities are restricted, and you regularly take one or two days off work at the time of your period.

You had a history of deep vein thrombosis while on the pill eighteen months ago. Your last cervical smear year ago was normal.

Past history: deep vein thrombosis (DVT)

Previous treatments: progestogens, mefenamic acid, Cyclokapron

Family history: nil

Social history: smokes twenty cigarettes/day; drinks ten units alcohol/week

Patient's attitude: fed up, heard about new operation that can cure her problem without needing hysterectomy

Examiner Instructions

Candidate will have fifteen minutes to take a history and discuss investigations and treatments. He or she may ask about the result of examination and your reply that there were no abnormalities. Use the below key to score:

Marking Sheet

A) Introduction

    Nonmedical language

    Eye contact

    Listen to patient

    Invites questions

                                            0   1   2   3   4   5

B) History

    Symptoms, duration, menstrual history

    Oral contraceptive pills (OCP)/DVT

    Sterilisation

    Medical treatment

Obstetric history

Social history

0 1 2 3 4 5

C) Investigations

Hemoglobin (Hb), iron studies

Hysteroscopy/biopsy

Ultrasound (US)

Thyroid function tests

Explanation of tests

0 1 2 3 4 5

D) Treatment

Ablation, resection

Mirena coil

Explanation

Risks/benefits

0 1 2 3 4 5

Discussion

Heavy menstrual bleeding (HMB) is defined as excessive menstrual blood loss that interferes with a woman's physical, social, emotional, and/or material quality of life. It can occur alone or in combination with other symptoms.

The *NHS Annual Evidence Update on Heavy Menstrual Bleeding: Examination and Investigations for 2009* advises that a woman should be sent for an ultrasound (US) investigation if

- the uterus is palpable abdominally,

- pelvic examination reveals a mass of uncertain origin, or

- medical treatment has failed.

It is very important that the person performing the scan is appropriately trained, or misleading results may be obtained."

Evidence from two reviews shows that ultrasound is an accurate method for identifying pathology (sensitivity 48–100 percent and specificity 12–100 percent). Furthermore, studies show that ultrasound is better at identifying fibroids than is hysteroscopy but is less accurate for identifying polyps or endometrial disease when compared with hysteroscopy. However, it is associated with higher completion rates (88 percent) and greater acceptability with women (11 percent finding it "unpleasant") when compared to a hysteroscopy (77 percent and 27 percent, respectively). Saline infusion sonography is an accurate method for identification of pathology, with a sensitivity of 85–100 percent and a specificity of 50–100 percent. One review found that for hysteroscopy the sensitivity was 90–97 percent, and the specificity was 62–93 percent. Hysteroscopy should be used as a diagnostic tool only when ultrasound results are inconclusive; for example, to determine the exact location of a fibroid or the exact nature of the abnormality.

In the early 1990s, it was estimated that at least 60 percent of women presenting with HMB went on to have a hysterectomy. This was often the only treatment offered. Hysterectomy is a major operation and is associated with significant complications in a minority of cases. Since the 1990s the number of hysterectomies has been decreasing rapidly.

If history and investigations indicate that pharmaceutical treatment is appropriate and either hormonal or nonhormonal treatments are acceptable, treatments should be considered in the following order:

o   levonorgestrel-releasing intrauterine system (LNG-IUS) provided long-term (at least twelve months) use is anticipated

o   tranexamic acid or nonsteroidal anti-inflammatory drugs (NSAIDs) or combined oral contraceptives (COCs)

o   norethisterone (15 mg) daily from days five to twenty-six of the menstrual cycle, or injected long-acting progestogens.

If hormonal treatments are not acceptable to the woman, then either tranexamic acid or NSAIDs can be used.

Endometrial ablation should be considered in women with HMB who have a normal uterus and also those with small uterine fibroids (less than 3 cm in diameter). In women with HMB alone, with uterus no bigger than a ten-week pregnancy, endometrial ablation should be considered preferable to hysterectomy. All women considering endometrial ablation should have access to a second-generation ablation technique. Second-generation ablation techniques should be used where no structural or histological abnormality is present. The second-generation techniques recommended for consideration are as follows. Providers should ensure that when purchasing any of these that they buy the least expensive available option.

Hysterectomy should not be used as a first-line treatment solely for HMB. Hysterectomy should be considered only when

- other treatment options have failed, are contraindicated, or are declined by the woman

- there is a wish for amenorrhoea;

- the woman (who has been fully informed) requests it; and

- the woman no longer wishes to retain her uterus and fertility.

Women offered hysterectomy should have a full discussion of the implication of the surgery before a decision is made. The discussion should include sexual feelings, fertility impact, bladder function, need for further treatment, treatment complications, the woman's expectations, alternative surgery, and psychological impact. Women offered hysterectomy should be informed about the increased risk of serious complications (such as intraoperative haemorrhage or damage to other abdominal organs) associated with hysterectomy when uterine fibroids are present.

Women should be informed about the risk of possible loss of ovarian function and its consequences, even if their ovaries are retained during hysterectomy. Individual assessment is essential when deciding the route of hysterectomy. The following factors need to be taken into account:

- presence of other gynaecological conditions or disease

- uterine size

- presence and size of uterine fibroids

- mobility and descent of the uterus

- size and shape of the vagina

- history of previous surgery

Taking into account the need for individual assessment, the route of hysterectomy should be considered in the following order: first-line vaginal; second-line abdominal. Under circumstances such as morbid obesity or the need for oophorectomy during vaginal hysterectomy, the laparoscopic approach should be considered, and appropriate expertise sought. When abdominal hysterectomy is decided upon, then both the total method

(removal of the uterus and the cervix) and subtotal method
(removal of the uterus and preservation of the cervix) should be
discussed with the woman.

Reference

NICE Clinical Guidelines CG44, "Heavy Menstrual Bleeding," 2007.

Gynaecology OSCE Station

Abnormal Cervical Smear

Candidate Instructions

Miss Sarah Jones is a twenty-two-year-old student who has been referred for colposcopy, as her smear test has been reported as showing severe dyskaryosis.

Miss Jones is very anxious and frightened and is refusing to have the examination.

You must explain the procedure to her and why it is important to try to have the examination today.

Role-Player Information

You are twenty-two-year-old student. You have just had your first smear test, and your GP has told you that you need to have a colposcopy. You think that you have cancer. After much persuasion by a friend, you have attended the colposcopy clinic with her. However, once the nurse explained the procedure to you, you are extremely scared and are refusing to have the examination.

You smoke twenty cigarettes/day and are sexually active. You have never been pregnant. Last menstrual period (LMP) 27 October, use the pill for contraception.

The candidate is expected to explain why you need a colposcopy. If the the candidate does not cover these points, you should ask direct questions regarding the following:

1) What smear test means and does not mean (e.g., regarding your having cancer or not).

Answer—the likelihood of *cervical intraepithelial neoplasia* CIN is 80–90 percent; likelihood of cancer of cervix is 5 percent and usually early stage.

2) Why you need the examination.

3) What the examination entails.

4) Biopsy (loop excision) will need to be taken, and result will be back in one week.

5) The biopsy is also treatment and is 95 percent successful.

6) The procedure can be performed under general anaesthesia (GA) but with increased risk.

7) Offer leaflets, counselling, and appointment next week.

Examiner Instruction

This patient has been misinformed about her cervical abnormalities, and the candidate must use his or her knowledge of national cervical screening programme guidelines to reassure her scientifically to calm her fears.

The candidate must explain in simple language the abnormality and the way it can be cured.

Marking Sheet

A) Counselling skills

Introduction

Eye contact

No jargons

Listen to patient/invite questions

Explain risk clearly

Explain options

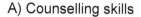

                  0 1 2 3 4 5 6 7 8 9 10

B) Knowledge

Explain the procedure

Why you need it

What is the most likely diagnosis/significance?

Risk of cancer

Need for biopsy/large loop excision of the transformation zone
(LLETZ)

Chance of cure

Sometimes GA needed

Follow-up and future smears

Leaflets   0 1 2 3 4 5 6 7 8 9 10

Discussion

Patients might often interpret precancerous cervical abnormalities
as cancer of the cervix, and patients need high standard of clarifi-
cation and a clear, simple leaflet to explain the implication of these
abnormalities.

Incidence and mortality rates in England have fallen considerably
over the past twenty years. During this period, incidence rates
decreased by over a third (from 15.0 to 9.8 per 100 000 female
population) and mortality rates reduced by 60 percent (from 5.8 to
2.2 per 100 000 female population in 2008 and 2009).

There were over 2 700 cervical cancer cases diagnosed in 2009
and around 750 deaths from cervical cancer in 2010.

The Cervical Screening Programme (CSP) aims to reduce the number of women who go on to develop cervical cancer by detecting and
treating preinvasive disease that may otherwise lead to cancer.

Incidence fell sharply following the establishment of the CSP in 1988, but this reduction has slowed in recent years. Between 2008 and 2009, there was a marked increase (14 percent) in the incidence of cervical cancer from 8.5 to 9.8 per 100 000 female population. This is likely to be due to earlier detection of cancers linked to increased screening coverage, particularly in women who may never have had a smear or not attended regularly for cervical screening. This increased screening coverage was a result of the media attention around the diagnosis.

The national CSP in the UK has very comprehensive guidelines and protocol of management and employment of national call and recall system.

Human papillomavirus (HPV) infection and its association with cervical cancer is now a well-known fact; those who have had early sex or many sexual partners are especially at risk of this.

However, most women who are infected with HPV do not go on to develop cervical cancer. Other factors that make it more difficult for the immune system or cells in the cervix to fight off the infection may also need to be present factors, such as smoking and immunosuppressant illnesses such as HIV/AIDS. In terms of early onset of sexual activity, HPV is not the only factor.

Research suggests that pregnancy before the age of seventeen, compared to having a first pregnancy at the age of twenty-five or over, doubles the risk of cervical cancer.

Menstrual Dysfunction

Gynaecology OSCE Station

Candidate Instructions

The GP has sent you this letter:

Dear Doctor,

I would like to refer to you this patient who is twenty-six years old with five years' history of heavy periods. She is getting very desperate, and now she is asking me to refer her to you in order to have a hysterectomy.

1) How you going to counsel her?

2) What are the alternatives to hysterectomy in her case?

3) When do you decide she needs a hysterectomy?

Examiner Instructions

Miss B is a twenty-six years old, para zero, and known to have eight years history of menorrhagia. Ever since she started menarche at the age of sixteen, she suffered from heavy periods with flooding. Her period used to last up to ten days in one stretch of heavy fresh loss with clots. To start with she used nonhormonal medications such as mefenamic and tranexaminic acid. This worked for few months and then stopped working.

After that she tried progestogens, both tablets and Provera injection. They as well worked for limited period of time. Last she was fitted a Mirena intrauterine system (IUS) which caused her very troublesome intermenstrual spotting and necessitated removal after a few months. Her last haemoglobin result was 7.2 g/dl. She needed three units of blood transfusion just fourteen days ago. She is very upset and exasperated, and she feels her life is not worth living.

Marking Sheet

1) How you going to counsel her?

History

Examination (general, abdominal, pelvic)

Full blood count (FBC), pelvic scan, liver function test (LFT), urea and electrolysis (U&E), clotting

Reasons for request

Pros and cons of hysterectomy   0 1 2 3 4 5

2) What are the alternatives to hysterectomy in her case? (ten marks)

GnRH—three monthly injection for eighteen months

Endometrial resection

Radiofrequency ablation

Laser ablation   0 1 2 3 4 5 6 7 8 9 10

3) When do you decide she needs a hysterectomy?

• Hysterectomy should not be used as a first-line treatment solely for menorrhagia.

• When other treatment options have failed, are contraindicated, or are declined.

• The patient's wish is to have amenorrhoea.

• The patient (who has been fully informed) requests it.

• The patient no longer wishes to retain her uterus and fertility.

                                          0 1 2 3 4 5

Discussion

This is a young patient who has had a very bad time with her periods since her menarche. She has never been investigated fully and never been counselled for implications of her condition on her life and living. Basically she was traumatised by her bad experience and has to be handled with care and by an experienced gynaecologist.

From the start she must be well informed about her condition, with full physiological and anatomical illustrations, and offered psychological support and counselling.

After comprehensive investigations to rule out any organic causes, including haematological investigations to role out any coagulation factors defect, she should be informed about other means to deal with her periods in order to avoid drastic intervention and possible associated complications short- and long-term. Down regulation and add back with GnRh and hormone replacement add back could be considered for a year or two to give her a real relief of her symptoms, which will have impact on her mental state. First- or second-generation endometrial ablation and resection must be considered.

In case of failure of these secondary measures, you have to put out a plan for further counselling for future fertility and when to consider hysterectomy with surrogate treatment.

Reference

NICE Clinical Guideline 44: "Heavy Menstrual Bleeding."

Subfertility Station

Gynaecology OSCE Station

Candidate Instructions

Mrs. and Mr. H. are sitting opposite you in a general gynaecology clinic. They been referred because of inability to conceive for over five years.

Part 1

1) How you going to assess them?

2) What specific investigations you will send off?

3) In a follow-up visit, you discover that there is an element of poor ovulation; what are the options available for treatment?

Part 2

Mrs. H. had a six-months programme of induction of ovulation, but she is not pregnant yet.

1- What is your further action?

2- She is getting very agitated, and the whole thing is affecting her marriage right now.

Examiner Instructions

Mrs. H. is thirty-three years old, para zero, and has been trying for a baby for five years without success. She has not consulted any medical advice before and was only self-treating with herbs and alternative medicine. Her menstrual history is of very irregular cycles since the age of sixteen. She never paid much attention to that, and she is kind of happy to have it that way. There is no previous medical or surgical history of notice, and she is taking only folic acid. Her BMI is 31 kg/m2, and she stopped smoking a few months ago in order to increase her chances of conception. She described having unprotected sexual intercourse at least three times/week over the last few years.

Mr H. is twenty-eight years old, never fathered any children before, had mumps at the age of four, but is otherwise healthy and fit, without a history of any medical or surgical problems. His BMI is 26 kg/m2, he smokes eight cigarettes/day, and he drinks alcohol socially.

1) How you going to assess them?

Menstrual history   01 2

Sexual history   01

Medical and surgical history   01

Social history   0 1

Drug history   01

Examination   01

BMI   0 1

2) What specific investigations you will send off?

Semen analysis   0 1 2 3

Day 21 progesterone   0 1

Pelvic scan   0 1 2

HSG   0 1 2

Hormonal profile   0 1

Rubella immunity   0 1

3) In a follow-up visit, you discovered that there is an element of poor ovulation; what are the options available for treatment?

Weight reduction   0 1

Clomiphene citrate   0 1 2

Metformin   0 1 2

Combination   0 1 2

Laparoscopic ovarian drilling   0 1 2

Gonadotrophins   0 1

Counselling   0 1

OSCE Station

Fertility 2

Candidate Instruction

A twenty-nine-year-old woman has been investigated for three years for primary infertility and found to have the following:

HSG	Patent tubes, normal uterine cavity
Day 21 S. progesterone	19 pmole/L
FSH	24 u/L
luteinizing hormone (LH)	35 u/L
S. prolactin	850 m unit/L

Semen analysis of her partner showed the following:

Count	20.7 M/ml
Motility	A—35%, B—20%
Morphology	10% normal form, 90% head defect
MAR	5% positive

She was put on clomiphene citrate for induction of ovulation and had four months of treatment.

Day 12 follicular tracking scan showed the scan pictures below:

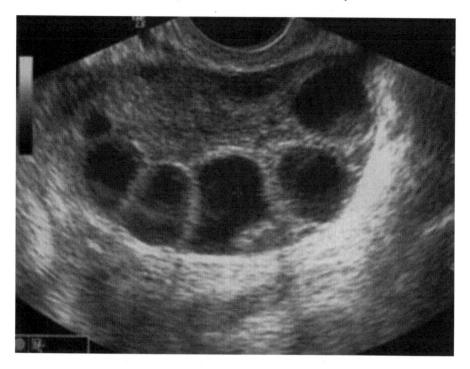

Figure 8: Transvaginal Scan (Google Images)

Advise her on the next step.

Plan her future management.

Examiner's Instructions

This is a case of primary infertility due to anovulation, candidate should show ability to take full history and highlight aspect of fertility investigations. He/she should explain the interpretation of individual test and plan stages of treatment.

Marking Sheet

Candidate should recognize the abnormal hormone profile and anovulatory s. progesterone.

0 1 **2 marks**

Candidate should confirm the normality of semen analysis.

0 1 **2 marks**

Candidate should read the scan and identify endometrium thickness of 12.1 mm, and there are three mature follicles.

0 1 2 marks

Candidate should advise the patient on implication of getting pregnant this month, and she might have multiple pregnancies.

0 1 2 marks

Candidate should plan her next treatment plan: continue on induction of ovulation, and reduce the clomiphene dosage.

0 1 2 marks

If she is not pregnant after four months of induction of ovulation, she should be advised to go for assisted conception.

0 1 2 3 4 marks

She should be told about the availability of IVF under the NHS, and she is entitled to have full funding.

0 1 2 3 4 marks

She must be counselled for treatment and to check the welfare of the child, and pre IVF investigation, such as for HIV and hepatitis are required for both her and her partner.

0 1 2 marks

Discussion

Couples who experience problems in conceiving should be seen together, because both partners are affected by decisions surrounding investigation and treatment.

History-taking in this case should involve full social, sexual, gynaecological, obstetrics, surgical, and medical histories and should be obtained with care and a sympathetic and gentle approach. Certain aspects of this section might give a clue to the cause of infertility.

People who experience fertility problems should be offered counselling because of the fertility problems themselves. The investigations and treatments of fertility problems can cause psychological stress. Counselling should be offered before, during, and after investigation and treatment, irrespective of the outcome of these procedures. Counselling should be provided by someone who is not directly involved in the management of the individual's and/or couple's fertility problems.

Preliminary investigation of this couple showed normal semen analysis as per (World Health Organization) WHO guidelines. However, the female investigation showed anovulation and slightly elevated Prolactin. In this situation, the day 21 s. progesterone as well as prolactin level should be repeated before embarking on induction of ovulations.

Ovulation disorders

Classification of ovulatory disorders

The WHO classifies ovulation disorders into three groups:

- Group I: hypothalamic pituitary failure (hypothalamic amenorrhoea or hypogonadotrophic hypogonadism)

- Group II: hypothalamic-pituitary-ovarian dysfunction (predominately polycystic ovary syndrome)

- Group III: ovarian failure

WHO Group I ovulation disorders

Advise women with WHO Group I anovulatory infertility that they can improve their chance of regular ovulation, conception, and an uncomplicated pregnancy by

- increasing their body weight if they have a BMI of less than 19, and/or

- moderating their exercise levels if they undertake high levels of exercise.

Offer women with WHO Group I ovulation disorders pulsatile administration of gonadotrophin-releasing hormone or gonadotrophins with luteinising hormone activity to induce ovulation.

In women with WHO Group II ovulation disorders receiving first-line treatment for ovarian stimulation: Advise women with WHO Group II anovulatory infertility who have a BMI of 30 or over to lose weight (see NICE recommendation 1.2.6.3). Inform them that this alone may restore ovulation, improve their response to ovulation induction agents, and have a positive impact on pregnancy outcomes. Offer women with WHO Group II anovulatory infertility one of the following treatments, taking into account potential adverse effects, ease and mode of use, the woman's BMI, and monitoring needed:

- clomiphene citrate, *or*

- metformin, *or*

- a combination of the above.

For women who are taking clomiphene citrate, offer ultrasound monitoring during at least the first cycle of treatment to ensure that they are taking a dose that minimises the risk of multiple pregnancy and ensures unifollicular ovulation.

For women who are taking clomiphene citrate, do not continue treatment for longer than six months.

Women prescribed metformin should be informed of the side effects associated with its use (such as nausea, vomiting, and other gastrointestinal disturbances).

For women with WHO Group II ovulation disorders who are known to be resistant to clomiphene citrate, consider one of the following second-line treatments, depending on clinical circumstances and the woman's preference:

- laparoscopic ovarian drilling, *or*

- combined treatment with clomiphene citrate and metformin if not already offered as first-line treatment, *or*

- gonadotrophins.

Women with *polycystic ovary syndrome* who are being treated with gonadotrophins should not be offered treatment with gonadotrophin-releasing hormone agonist concomitantly, because it does not improve pregnancy rates, and it is associated with an increased risk of ovarian hyperstimulation.

The use of adjuvant growth hormone treatment with gonadotrophin-releasing hormone agonist and/or human menopausal gonadotrophin during ovulation induction in women with polycystic ovary syndrome who do not respond to clomiphene citrate is not recommended, because it does not improve pregnancy rates.

The effectiveness of pulsatile gonadotrophin-releasing hormone in women with clomiphene citrate-resistant polycystic ovary syndrome is uncertain and is therefore not recommended outside a research context.

Clomiphene induction of ovulation must be monitored closely with ovarian follicular tracking by transvaginal scan (TVS) to confirm the follicular maturation, time the human chorionic gonadotrophin (HCG) injection to trigger ovulation, and adjust the dose to improve response to the treatment and prevent multiple birth.

Referral for assisted conception is the next step up to improve pregnancy rate; although IUI does improve the pregnancy rate, some doctors do not recommend IUI and prefer to go directly for IVF.

Independent counselling by a well-qualified fertility councillor is mandatory, and full investigation and pre-IVF investigation must be undertaken before assisted conception.

Gynaecology OSCE Station

Uterine Fibroids

Candidate Instructions

A thirty-five-year-old woman with uterine fibroid and heavy period is presented to you at the gynaecology clinic and wishes to discuss her treatment with you. She has been trying to get pregnant for four years. She was told during her last operation that her tubes were patent.

After telling her about hysterectomy, myomectomy, and uterine artery embolisation, take the following steps:

1) Please take a full history.

2) Consider how you are going to investigate this patient to help you on planning her treatment.

3) Discuss the risk(s) you might encounter during her management.

Examiner Instructions

This thirty-five-year-old woman has been suffering very much from heavy and prolonged and painful periods interfering with her job and relationship. She had two previous laparotomies and myomectomies for multiple fibroids: the first was in Nigeria four years ago; the second was in the UK last year, when ten fibroids were removed, and she was told that her tubes and ovaries were normal.

She is keen on getting pregnant, but her priority is to get better and to improve her living.

Her husband is forty years old and has no children and was investigated four years ago and found to have normal semen analysis.

She was told that she might lose her uterus if she will need a third myomectomy; she does not mind considering adoption if she had to have a hysterectomy.

Marking Sheet

3- Full gynaecological history　　　　　　0 1 2 3 4 5 6 marks

　　Previous investigations into fertility

　　Complications during and after the previous operations

　　Full menstrual history and effect of pain and bleeding on day-to-day living

　　Previous measures to manage her period problems

General examination and abdominal and pelvic evaluation

2- Evaluation of her condition   0 1 2 3 4 5 6 marks

Size and mobility of fibroids

Haemoglobin electrophoresis

Pelvic and abdominal scan

Magnetic resonance imaging (MRI) abdomen and pelvis

HSG

3- As part of her comprehensive informed consent, she opted for myomectomy; the risks encountered include the following:

                                        0 1 2 3 4 5 6 7 8

Primary perioperative bleeding

Injuries to bladder and bowels

Need for hysterectomy

Postoperative bleeding and return to theatre

Discussion

This patient with primary infertility and two previous myomectomies is at high risk of complications during any surgical intervention to deal with her fibroids.

The couple must be warned that further myomectomy could lead to loss of her uterus as a result of uncontrolled bleeding during and/or after surgery and might need further intervention to deal with complications. Patient must be informed about other means of achieving fertility (e.g., adoption or surrogacy).

Uterine artery embolisation (UAE) must be discussed: patient should be informed about her suitability for such a procedure, and the following information should be discussed:

1-Conservative treatment is offered including UAE.

2-UAE is not recommended for woman who wish to maintain fertility.

3- UAE may improve bleeding related complains in about 75–90 percent.

4- The risk of developing menopause after intervention is the same in all surgical intervention and UAE.

5-Treatment is not always needed to deal with multiple uterine fibroids.

6-Ultrasound is the imaging modality of choice in the detection and evaluation of uterine fibroids.

7-The less invasive nature of UAE needs to be balanced against the need for reintervention in almost a third of patients.

Further Discussion

Uterine fibroids are classified as either intramural (if they had less than 50 percent protrusion into the serosal surface) or sub-serosal (if they had >50% protrusion into the serosal surface, or submucosal, if they protrude into the endometrial cavity. This later group divided into Grade 0, 1, or 2, depending on degree of protrusion into the uterine cavity and the angle they form with the endometrium.

Among women who underwent removal of submucosal fibroids, the live birth rate jumped from 23 percent before surgery to 52 percent after surgery.

Malignant leiomyosarcomas are rare and can arise de novo.

Rarely, uterine leiomyomas may undergo malignant degeneration to become sarcomas. The true incidence of malignant transforma-tion is difficult to determine, because leiomyomas are common, whereas malignant leiomyosarcomas are rare and can arise de novo. The incidence of malignant degeneration is less than 1.0 percent.

Calcified fibroids are often depicted on conventional radiographs of the pelvis. In some patients, an MRI provides additional information. The role of computed tomography (CT) scanning is limited. Calcifications may be more visible on CT scans than on conventional radiographs because of the superior contrast differentiation achieved with CT scanning.

MRI has an important role in defining the anatomy of the uterus and ovaries, as well as in assessing disease in patients in whom US findings are confusing. MRI also may be helpful in planning myomectomy or selective surgical removal of a fibroid.

OSCE Station

Urogynaecology station

Candidate Instructions

You are a registrar in the gynaecology clinic; your consultant urogynaecologist asks you to see the last patient for him.

Referral Letter

Dear Doctor:

This 46-year-old woman has experienced urinary incontinence for many years, which is getting worse. She does not suffer from any other problems, and vaginal examination revealed no vaginal prolapse. She is overweight, but her weight is steady. She has not had a period for months, and gonadotrophins indicate menopausal levels. She finds that her leakage is distressing, especially when playing her favourite netball game. She is keen to explore the possibility of surgery to help with her urinary incontinence, having previously found pelvic floor exercises to be of no benefit. I am grateful to your help with further assessment with view to this.

Part 1

1- Take a full history.

2- Plan her investigations.

3- How are you going to plan her management?

Part 2

Review the urodynamic study, explain the finding to Mrs. J. G., and inform her about the plan of her management.

Figure 8: Uroflowmetry

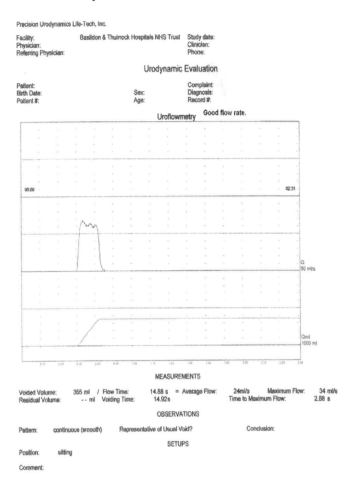

Precision Urodynamics Life-Tech, Inc.

Facility:	Basildon & Thurrock Hospitals NHS Trust	Study date:
Physician:		Clinician:
Referring Physician:		Phone:

Urodynamic Evaluation

Patient:			Complaint:
Birth Date:		Sex:	Diagnosis:
Patient #:		Age:	Record #:

Uroflowmetry   Good flow rate.

MEASUREMENTS

Voided Volume:	355 ml	/ Flow Time:	14.88 s	= Average Flow:	24ml/s	Maximum Flow:	34 ml/s
Residual Volume:	-- ml	Voiding Time:	14.92s			Time to Maximum Flow:	2.88 s

OBSERVATIONS

Pattern: continuous (smooth)   Representative of Usual Void?   Conclusion:

SETUPS

Position: sitting

Comment:

20/11/2012   15:15:13   PVR = Post Void Residual

95

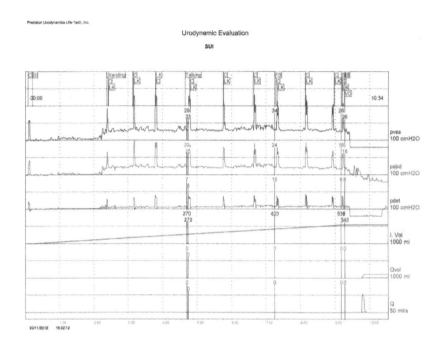

Figure 9: Urodynamic Study

Examiner Instruction

This patient has been complaining of stress incontinence for many years and getting worse recently, especially when playing netball. She denied any urgency or urge incontinence, and vaginal examination did not show any vaginal prolapse. She had her menopause eight months ago. She had a history of abnormal cervical smear, but the most recent smears are normal. She has two children delivered with normal vaginal delivery; both babies were large birth weight—4.1 kg and 4.3 kg—and had some urinary dysfunction for a short period after birth and was corrected after intense pelvic-muscles exercises.

She was doing an input and output chart for nearly one week, and her recent midstream urine (MSU) was normal. Pelvic ultrasound showed normal pelvic organs.

Her recent urodynamics showed stable bladder, no evidence of high residual volume, and maximum bladder volume of 350 ml. She demonstrated leakage on coughing and straining.

She is well informed about the minimal access surgery for treatment of stress incontinence.

Marking Sheet

Gynaecological and bladder dysfunction history

Menstrual history

Cervical cytology

Urinary incontinence, frequency, urgency, stress, and overactive bladder (OAB)

Bowel dysfunction   0 1 2 3 4 5

Obstetrics history

Parity and method of delivery

Birth weight

Postdelivery bladder dysfunction   0 1 2 3

Examination

    Abdomen for full bladder and abdominal mass

    Neurological perineal examination

Pelvic and vaginal examination   0 1 2 3 4 5

    Investigations

    Bladder diary

    MSU

    Pelvic and abdominal scan

    Urodynamics   0 1 2 3 4

    Planning her treatment in view of her above findings

    Weight reduction

    Continue pelvic muscles exercises

    Tension-free vaginal tape obturator (TVTO)   0 1 2 3

Discussion

History-taking of women with urinary incontinence (UI) or OAB guides the investigation and management by evaluating symptoms, their progression, and the impact of symptoms on lifestyle. .

Taking a history also allows the assessment of risk factors associated with the possible diagnoses. The relevant elements of history follow

History-taking is regarded as the cornerstone of assessment of UI. Current practice is that women with UI are categorised according to their symptoms into those with stress, mixed, or urgency UI; women with mixed UI are treated according to the symptom they report to be the most troublesome. In the absence of evidence that urodynamic testing improves the outcome of women treated conservatively, and without robust evidence that urodynamic testing provides additional valuable information to the history alone in the initial assessment of women with UI, the NICE guidelines concluded that urodynamic testing is not required before initiating conservative treatment.

Obstetric and Gynaecological History

The number and type of deliveries and their outcome would normally be documented. The woman's desire for further childbearing should also be established, as this may have implications for the most appropriate treatment options. The menstrual history and menopausal status should be determined and enquiry made into symptoms of uterovaginal prolapse. The woman's sexual function and her expectations from this point of view should also be considered.

In order to reach a clinical diagnosis, a urinary history is taken to determine storage and voiding patterns and symptoms. The major symptoms to consider include the following:

• Storage symptoms:

- frequency (daytime), nocturia, urgency, urgency UI

- stress UI

- constant leakage (which may rarely indicate fistula)

• Voiding symptoms:

- hesitancy, straining to void, poor or intermittent urinary stream

• Postmicturition symptoms:

- sensation of incomplete emptying, postmicturition dribbling—
  accompanying symptoms may indicate the possibility of
  a more serious diagnosis that requires referral, such as
  haematuria, persisting bladder or urethral pain, or recurrent
  urinary tract infection (UTI), which can also be identified when
  taking a urinary history.

If a woman does not report mixed UI (i.e., if she reports pure stress
UI or pure urgency UI), the probability of finding urodynamic stress
incontinence (USI) plus detrusal overactivity(DO) on cystometry is
small (around 10 percent), therefore urodynamic testing might be
said to offer little additional diagnostic value. It is acknowledged
that urodynamic investigation is not simply used to distinguish
USI and DO, and that further information may be obtained about
other elements of lower urinary-tract function, such as the voiding
pattern.

If a woman does not report pure urgency UI, the probability of finding
DO on cystometry is small (again around 10 percent), therefore
urodynamic testing offers little added diagnostic value.

Physical Examination

Abdominal examination can detect a significantly enlarged bladder or palpable pelvic mass. A palpable bladder may indicate the presence of chronic urinary retention. Palpation may detect a volume of 300 ml or more. Urinary incontinence may occur in association with urinary retention (often called overflow incontinence).

Pelvic assessment is important and should include vaginal examination and possibly also rectal examination if clinically indicated. Vaginal examination can assess pelvic organ prolapse (POP) and identify atrophic changes, infection, and excoriation. Uterine and ovarian enlargement may be determined by bimanual examination. When rectal examination is undertaken, it is used to further evaluate posterior vaginal wall prolapse and, where indicated by a history of constipation, prolapse or faecal incontinence.

Neurophysiology

Neurophysiological tests include assessments of nerve conduction and electromyography (EMG). The former include sacral reflex latencies, pudendal terminal motor latencies, and evoked potentials, which test the integrity of nerve pathways relating to voiding and continence. Abnormal results might indicate underlying neurological dysfunction. Electromyography tests the end organ function of somatic muscles of the pelvic floor, or sphincter complexes, but cannot be used to record activity from smooth muscle. No evidence was identified that addressed diagnostic accuracy of neurophysiological testing in relation to idiopathic UI. Where history suggests evidence of neurological disease, examination of lower limbs together with sacral sensation and sacral reflexes is required.

Urinalysis is used to detect infection, protein, blood, and glucose in the urine. Protein may indicate infection and/or renal impairment, blood may indicate infection or malignancy, and glucose may indicate diabetes mellitus. Some findings on urine testing indicate referral.

Some findings on physical examination or from history-taking in relation to emptying may indicate referral because of suspected voiding dysfunction. Abdominal examination can detect a significantly enlarged bladder, which may indicate the presence of chronic urinary retention. Palpation may detect a volume of 300 ml or more. Large postvoid residual urine may indicate the presence of underlying bladder outlet obstruction, neurological disease, or detrusor failure. These would be a reason for referral to a specialist rather than progression through a path of conservative treatments. Large residual urine—in effect chronic retention of urine—may also present with renal failure, although this.

Bladder diaries are used to document each cycle of filling and voiding over a number of days and can provide information about urinary frequency, urgency, diurnal and nocturnal cycles, functional bladder capacity, and total urine output. They also record leakage episodes, fluid intake, and pad changes and give an indication of the severity of wetness. They may also be used for monitoring the effects of treatment.

The term "urodynamics" encompasses a number of varied physiological tests of bladder and urethral function, which aim to demonstrate an underlying abnormality of storage or voiding. The term is often used loosely to mean multichannel cystometry.

Cystometry is the measurement of intravesical pressure, which can be carried out through a single recording channel (simple cystometry) or, more commonly, by multichannel cystometry, which involves the synchronous measurement of both bladder and intra-abdominal pressures by means of catheters inserted into the bladder and the rectum or vagina. The aim is to replicate the woman's symptoms by filling the bladder and observing pressure changes or leakage caused by provocation tests.

Uroflowmetry entails a free-flow void into a recording device, which provides the practitioner with information about the volume of urine passed and the rate of urine flow.

There are also numerous tests of urethral function, including urethral pressure profilometry and leak-point pressure measurement. These are used to derive values that reflect the ability of the urethra to resist urine flow, expressed most commonly as maximum urethral closure pressure (MUCP) or as abdominal, cough, or Valsalva leak-point pressures (ALPP, CLPP, and VLPP, respectively).

Videourodynamics involves synchronous radiographic screening of the bladder with multichannel cystometry and is so called because originally the information was recorded to videotape. Ambulatory

OSCE Station

Amenorrhoea

Candidate Instruction

You are registrar in an infertility clinic; you have a new referral from a GP asking for further management.

GP Letter

Dear Doctor:

Thank you for seeing this couple for consideration for fertility treatment. Karen is a 38-year-old lady who had premature ovarian failure at the age of twenty-four years and was under the care of another hospital for secondary amenorrhoea. She was on HRT and subsequently lost to follow-up.

She was treated for CIN in 2003 when she had large loop excision of transformation zone (LLETZ).

She is cohabiting with Mr. P. H., whose semen analysis has shown teratospermia. Neither of them has children.

Many thanks.

Yours sincerely,

Dr. Paul Smith

Part 1

1- Take full gynaecological history.

2- Initiate some investigations.

3- What are your immediate measures?

Part 2

This lady is still amenorrhea, and her hormone profile is as follows:

E2	>18 pm/l
FSH	66 U/L
LH	28 U/L
PRL	145 mu/l

1- What action might you need to take immediately?

2—What is/are the line/s of management you should adopt, and what is your priority?

Examiner Instructions

This thirty-eight-year-old woman has had amenorrhoea since the age of twenty-four. She attained her menarche at the age of eleven and had irregular periods. She went on the pill for one year and came off it at the age of twenty-four, and since then she has had no spontaneous periods.

She was investigated at her local district general hospital and was referred to a tertiary centre for further evaluation. After many investigations she was told that she has premature ovarian failure (POF) and has to go on HRT.

She took continuous combined hormone replacement therapy (CCHRT) for a short period of time (four years) and was informed by a doctor to stop HRT to avoid breast cancer. She felt joint pain and was feeling weak and tired and has been to her GP, who suggested to her to go for a dual energy X-ray absorptiometry (DEXA) scan to check her bone mineral density (BMD). The DEXA scan for BMD showed osteoporosis. She was commenced on bisphosphonate for two years. Yearly BMD scan showed improvement to osteopenia. The last DEXA scan was three years ago, and she is not on any replacement of bone-building medication.

She has been having mild vasomotor symptoms and feeling tired. She has had treatment for CIN with LLETZ in 2003, and her smears are normal. Last cervical smear was 2013 and was negative.

She has another sister who requires IVF treatment for male factor. She has no family history of POF or any chromosomal abnormalities.

Her recent scan showed the following:

Small uterine body.

Endometrium 4.3 mm.

Both ovaries are small, and there were no follicles seen.

Marking Sheet

Gynaecological history

    Period irregularity

    Age of menarche

    History of abnormal cervical smear   0 1 2 3

Family history   0 1 2

Initial investigations

    Hormone profile

    Baseline scan

    DEXA scan   0 1 2 3 4

Management priority

    Hormone replacement therapy

    IVF with egg donation

    Yearly BMD with DEXA scan   0 1 2 3 4

Discussion

This patient is a case of POF; she was started with premature ovarian insufficiency (POI) masked by going on the pill
and followed by another delay of diagnosis because of postpill
amenorrhoea. The diagnosis was realized only after prolonged
amenorrhoea and appropriate investigations after tertiary referral.
She was on hormone replacement but came off after inappropri-
ate advice. She was without HRT for number of years; ultimately
a BMD study showed osteoporosis, and she was then started on
bisphosphonate. For two years after this she was lost to follow-up.

Her last BMD study was three years ago, and she was off the HRT
for nearly six years. She suffers from vasomotor symptom and weak-
ness and tiredness. She declined to go on cyclical HRT, because she
does not like to start having a period; therefore, she was started on
continuous combined hormone replacement therapy (CCHRT). Her
main problem is oestrogen depletion and fertility management.

Premature ovarian failure refers to a loss of normal function of the
ovaries before the age of forty.

Premature ovarian failure is sometimes referred to as premature
menopause, but the two conditions are not exactly the same.
Women with premature ovarian failure—also known as primary
ovarian insufficiency—may have irregular or occasional periods
for years and may even become pregnant. Women with premature
menopause stop having periods and can't become pregnant.

Restoring oestrogen levels in women with premature ovarian failure helps prevent some complications, such as osteoporosis, but infertility is harder to treat.

- *Premature ovarian failure* is the extreme state of complete primordial follicle depletion. This is an irreversible state characterized by the presence of amenorrhea, permanent infertility, and elevated menopausal gonadotrophin levels. At present no proven method can determine that a woman has no primordial follicles remaining in the ovary, so, in effect, this term is merely a construct (i.e., a concept that cannot be proven). For this reason, the authors prefer not to use the term premature ovarian failure (POF).

Aging is associated with a decline in the number of ovarian follicles, menstrual irregularities, ovarian hormonal deficiency, anovulation, decreased fertility, and finally a complete and irreversible cessation of menses, known as menopause, usually occurring at a mean age of fifty-one years.

Ovarian Clinical Situation	Menses	Gonadotrophins	Fertility
Occult insufficiency	Normal	Normal	Reduced
Biochemical insufficiency	Abnormal	Elevated	Reduced
Overt insufficiency	Abnormal	Elevated	Reduced
Premature ovarian failure	Absent	Elevated	Zero

Follicle Depletion

Follicle depletion is a major pathogenetic mechanism for development of POI/POF.

The presence of normal numbers of follicles in the ovaries (approximately 300 000–400 000 at the beginning of puberty) is crucial for normal periodic ovulation. Full maturation of one dominant follicle is dependent on the simultaneous development of a support cohort of nondominant follicles. These, although destined to undergo atresia, play an important role in the fine-tuning of the hypothalamic-pituitary-ovarian axis by secreting regulatory hormones such as estradiol, inhibins, activins, and androgens.

Pathological conditions that cause depletion or a reduction of the follicle number may lead to a disruption of the highly coordinated process of follicular growth and ovulation. The lack of developing follicles leads to reduced circulating estradiol and inhibin levels and elevated serum FSH and LH. Occasionally, a "lonely" follicle may develop, stimulated by the high levels of FSH; however, instead of progressing to a normal ovulation, it is inappropriately luteinized (by the high LH levels) and may persist as a cystic structure visible on ultrasonography.

The ovarian follicle reserve can be depleted prematurely because of a low initial number or an accelerated rate of follicle atresia.

Low initial number.

- A disruption in any step of germ-cell formation, migration, oogonia proliferation, and meiosis results in a deficient initial follicle number. The final outcome could be a formation of streak gonads and primary amenorrhea, as in familial 46, XX gonadal dysgenesis, an autosomal-dominant disease with sex-linked inheritance.

- In milder cases, the initial follicle number is sufficient to support pubertal development, initiation of menstrual cycles, and even fertility, but ovarian failure due to follicle depletion develops early in the reproductive life.

- In primates, the foetal thymus plays an important role in establishing the normal endowment of primordial follicles. Not surprisingly, human conditions with thymic hypoplasia/aplasia have been associated with POI/POF.

Accelerated follicle atresia

Accelerated follicle atresia or destruction can result from one of the following:

- X chromosome monosomy/aneuploidy or mosaicism (as observed in Turner syndrome or some cases with 47, XXX karyotype)

- X chromosome abnormalities (X chromosome rearrangement, X isochromosome and ring chromosome, translocations of X chromosome material to an autosome [t(X;A)], fragile X premutation)

- Galactosaemia

- Cytotoxic therapy

- Irradiation

- Inflammation

The genes and chromosome regions implicated in the development of POI/POF are as follows:

- X chromosome genes: Multiple X chromosome genes are involved in regulating female fertility and reproductive lifespan and may be involved in the pathogenesis of ovarian failure.

  o Xp (short arm) genes: Deletions or disruptions of critical regions of the short arm of the X chromosome (Xp11, Xp22.1–21.3) have been described in association with gonadal dysgenesis and primary or secondary amenorrhea. The importance of the genes located on the short arm of the X chromosome for normal ovarian development, and survival is evident from the fact that half the patients with partial deletions of the short arm of the X chromosome have amenorrhea.

    - *Zfx* (X-linked zinc finger protein): Located on Xp22.1–21.3, this gene encodes a widely expressed protein of unknown function. *Zfx* "knockout" mice are small, less fertile, and have a diminished germ-cell number in the ovaries and testes.

    - *USP9X* gene (ubiquitin-specific protease 9 gene): It is located on Xp11.4, and its product is widely expressed in many tissues. In *Drosophila,* USP9X is required for eye development and oogenesis, but its role in human gonadal development is unclear.

  o Xq (long arm) genes: Analysis of terminal deletions and autosomal translocations yielded information on the

112

importance of several areas located on the long arm of the X chromosome. These include Xq13–21, Xq22–25, and Xq26–28.

- *FMR1* gene: This gene is located on Xq27.3. Mutations in this gene represent expansions of CGG (cytosine-guanine-guanine) repeat in the promoter region of the *FMR1* gene. One to forty CGG repeats are considered normal, forty to sixty repeats are considered a grey area, sixty to two hundred repeats are considered premutation, and more than two hundred CGG repeats represent full mutation. Full mutation is associated with mental retardation, while women with premutation demonstrate a twenty to thirty times increased incidence of POI/POF and are not affected by mental retardation. Why women with the full mutation have no ovarian failure and only those with premutation have ovarian failure is unclear. This may be related to unusual increases in mRNA levels in premutation carriers.

- XIST locus (X inactivation site): Located on Xq13, this locus is required for the reactivation of the silenced X chromosome during oocyte maturation. Two X chromosomes with two intact XIST loci are necessary for normal meiosis to occur in oocytes. Thus, impairment of the XIST locus results in meiotic arrest and oocyte depletion due to apoptosis.

- *DIA* gene (diaphanous gene): This gene, located on Xq21, is homologous to the diaphanous gene in *Drosophila*. DIA protein is abundantly expressed in the ovaries and other tissues and is important

for establishing cell polarity and morphogenesis.
DIA mutations in *Drosophila* lead to sterility in both
sexes. The Xq21 region contains at least seven
other genes involved in ovarian development. This
region is pseudoautosomal (present on both X and Y
chromosomes).

- Autosomal abnormalities

  o Trisomies 13 and 18, but not trisomy 21, are associated
    with ovarian dysgenesis and failure. Therefore, a
    possibility exists that ovarian genes are located on
    chromosomes 13 and 18.

  o Balanced autosomal translocations have been found in
    otherwise healthy women with POI/POF.

  o 46, XX gonadal dysgenesis/agenesis

    ▪ Approximately two thirds of cases with gonadal
      dysgenesis in individuals who are 46, XX are genetic.
      The inheritance is autosomal recessive, and the
      penetrance is variable. Therefore, a possibility exists
      that some of the sporadic cases of karyotypically
      normal POI/POF could be due to a mutant somatic
      gene for XX gonadal dysgenesis.

    ▪ 46, XX gonadal dysgenesis sometimes is a part of
      a genetic syndrome, such as gonadal dysgenesis
      and neurosensory deafness (Perrault syndrome);
      gonadal dysgenesis and cerebellar ataxia; gonadal
      dysgenesis, arachnodactyly, and microcephaly; and

gonadal dysgenesis, short stature, and metabolic acidosis.

o   Autosomal recessive disorders associated with POI/POF include the following:

  ▪   Cockayne syndrome

  ▪   Nijmegen breakage syndrome

  ▪   Werner syndrome

  ▪   Bloom syndrome

o   *ATM* gene (ataxia-telangiectasia mental retardation gene)

  ▪   ATM is a protein kinase involved in DNA metabolism and cell cycle control.

  ▪   Mutations in this gene, located on chromosome 11q22–23, are associated with ovarian atrophy and amenorrhea despite normal female sexual differentiation.

SECTION 3

OBSTETRICS

OSCE Stations

Prioritisation of Labour Ward Board

Candidate Instructions

You are the registrar on labour ward; you started your shift at 08.30. There is no consultant obstetrician on labour ward, but one consultant in the clinic is ready to come if needed.

Can you please prioritise the following based on the information provided on the board.

You have the following staff and resources at your disposal.

1) Experienced SHO

2) Obstetric anaesthetic registrar

3) Midwife coordinator who can suture episiotomies and insert cannulae

4) One senior midwife

5) One junior midwife

Marks will be awarded for logically prioritising each room, putting in place a management plan, and using resources appropriately.

Room	Name	Parity	Gestation	VE & time	Comments
1	Sheila Smith	1	40+2	0.00 2 cm 04.0 3 cm	Membrane intact, previous fourth- degree tear
2	Geraldine Archer	2	36+1	08.00 9 cm, clear liquor	DCDA twins, twin 1 ceph, twin 2 breech
3	Sharmaine Fush	0	36+6	06.00 Closed os	Admitted 00.00 with antepartum haemorrage (APH); confirmed foetal death in utero
4	Shelly Lewis	1	40+5	Second prostin at 06.00	Induction of labour (IOL) for big baby

5	Stephanie Mark	0	39+4	8:00 5 cm	Late decelerations, baseline tachycardia
6	Grace Pinker	1	41+1	04.00 4 cm	Low risk
7	Harriet Hussain	9	37+6	07:00 7 cm	

Marking Sheet

Marks should be awarded for the clarity and correctness of decision-making. Two marks are awarded for each correct management and one mark awarded for correct prioritisation.

Rome 1; low priority

Patient has been in latent phase. She is due for reassessment; ARM should be considered at this point. She can be assigned to a midwife.

Room 2; intermediate priority

She may be soon approaching second stage. Consideration should be made for moving her to theatre for delivery. Check that she has IV access for regional anaesthesia. Check paediatric availability and confirm that anaesthetist is aware. She will need the obstetric registrar and a senior midwife.

Room 3; high priority

Patient needs to be reviewed and given her options for delivery of her dead baby. Give consideration to misoprostol/Prostin IOL, talk about post-mortem. Also she needs IV line, checking FBC and clotting.

Room 4; low priority

Patient needs re assessment at 12.00 for ARM +/- syntocinon or third Prostin. She can be assigned to junior midwife.

Room 5; high priority

She has pathological CTG.

She needs urgent assessment for either delivery or foetal blood sampling.

Room 6; low priority

Low risk, no immediate problems, can be assigned to a midwife.

Room 7; intermediate priority

Grand multipara; she needs active management of third stage of labour and experienced midwife. IV line and FBC.

Station 2

Risk Management

Candidate Instructions

You are the lead clinician in charge of labour ward, and you have recently reviewed a letter from the clinical risk manager.

Letter

Dear Sir:

It has recently come to my notice that the department received two letters of complaints from patients who have delivered in your labour ward within the last two months.

Both ladies had shoulder dystocia, one baby had a fractured clavicle, and the other had Erb's Palsy. One parent is editor of the local paper. I am sure you realise that this would not be good for the hospital reputation, not to mention the staff morale, if this parent chooses to go ahead with a lead article criticising the care she received. I appreciate your earliest suggestion regarding a suitable plan of action.

Yours sincerely,

John smith

<u>What would be your plan of action?</u>

Examiner Instructions

The purpose of this station is to test candidate's knowledge and understanding of clinical risk management (CRM).

Marking Sheet

What is CRM? It is a process of identifying and investigating cases where the perception of risk has arisen, which includes cases with poor outcome and near misses.   0 1 2 marks

In the first instance, the two cases need to be reviewed by lead clinician and delivery suite manager and statements requested from staff involved.   0 1 2 marks

CRM should analyse management in the two cases and establish if management was according to the unit protocol.

Assess if changes to existing protocol are needed.

Give feedback to the staff in a nonblaming environment.

Organise fire drills in managing shoulder dystocia.

Start off an audit on the management of shoulder dystocia, and analyse results after a set time to see if management has improved.

0 1 2 3 4 marks

Face-to-face meeting with the parents should be arranged in a relaxed setting to listen to them, see how they are coping, and answer their questions.

You should discuss the cases also with the paediatrician and ask about the likely recovery from injuries, and it is advisable to organise another meeting with parents in the presence of paediatrician.

You should be open with the parents by explaining to them the faults in their care, if any, and how you are dealing with that.

0 1 2 marks

OSCE Station

Respiratory Disease

Candidate Instruction

You are on call on labour ward and were asked by one of the midwives to review the lady in room 4. She told you a very brief report about her: primiparous at thirty-nine weeks' gestation, admitted three hours ago in early labour; now her pain getting worse, but she is also very short of breath, and her chest making funny noises.

1) What is your approach in dealing with the patient chest symptoms?

2) You made a diagnosis of acute severe asthma; how you going to manage her?

3) Her condition is deteriorating; what are you going to do?

Examiner Instructions

She is thirty-two years old, with a long history of asthma since the age of twenty. Before pregnancy her asthma ran a very variable course, with good and bad seasons. However, the last few years were particularly bad, with several admissions to accident and emergency unit with severe asthma attacks. One time she was admitted to ITU in view of the seriousness of her condition. In between attacks she was put on maintenance treatment with cromolyn tablets and inhaled triamcinolone.

Luckily enough this pregnancy went well, and in fact her asthma had improved while she continued the above medications.

She was undertaking serial foetal ultrasound scanning in view of her condition and also because the baby was growing on the low side (at the third centile).

Since the beginning of her pregnancy, she was very scared from the idea of vaginal delivery, and she requested to have elective caesarean section on several occasions. She was convinced lately to have a go and see how she copes and keep an open mind.

Marking Sheet

1) What is your approach in dealing with her complaint?

Pain control   0 1

History   0 1

Examination   0 1

Oxygen and maintain   0 1

High saturation

Anaesthetic opinion   0 1 2

2) You made a diagnosis of acute severe asthma; how you going to manage her?

Keep O2 sat > 95%   0 1

Inhaled beta agonist   0 1 2

Oral steroid   0 1 2

Systemic steroid   0 1 2

Reassess situation   0 1

3) Her condition is deteriorating; what are you going to do?

Consider delivery   0 1

Rule out preeclampsia   0 1

Rule out pulmonary oedema   0 1 2

Rule out pulmonary embolism   0 1 2

Exclude chest infection   0 1

Total score 20 = final score

14 = good pass, 9–11= pass, 6–8 = borderline, less than 5 = fail

Discussion

Research consistently shows that women with well-controlled asthma can have healthy pregnancies with excellent maternal and perinatal outcomes. The ultimate goal of controlling asthma during pregnancy is to ensure that the foetus continues to get adequate oxygen by preventing asthma attacks.

Because it is unknown how pregnancy will affect an individual woman's symptoms, lung function of women with persistent asthma should be monitored during pregnancy, using common pulmonary function parameters such as spirometry, the peak expiratory flow rate (PEFR), and forced expiratory volume in one second (FEV_1). If possible, first-trimester ultrasound should also be performed to assess foetal growth restriction and risk of pre-term birth. Starting at thirty-two weeks, ultrasound exams to monitor foetal activity and growth should be considered for women with poorly controlled asthma, moderate to severe asthma, or who are recovering from a severe asthma attack.

Avoiding allergens and irritants, such as tobacco smoke, that exacerbate asthma can improve maternal well-being and lessen the need for medication. Asthmatic women are advised to identify triggers and do what they can to reduce them at home. Specific measures to reduce mould, dust mite exposure, animal dander, cockroaches, and other environmental triggers may be necessary. If acid reflux stimulates their asthma, women may want to try solutions such as elevating the head of a bed, eating smaller meals, not eating within a few hours of bedtime, and avoiding foods that trigger reflux.

Many women with asthma need to use medication to maintain normal respiratory function. Long-term medications—such as inhaled corticosteroids—are used to prevent asthma flare-ups, while rescue therapy—most commonly inhaled short-acting beta agonists (preferably inhaled albuterol during pregnancy)—provide immediate relief from symptoms. Whatever therapy is used, it should be tailored to supply pregnant patients with the lowest dose necessary to control their asthma.

Women who already use immunotherapy (allergy shots) at or near maintenance level to improve asthma symptoms may continue getting shots during pregnancy. However, women should not begin immunotherapy during pregnancy. Allergy shots are typically given with lower doses of serum to start and then are gradually increased to higher levels. These escalating doses may cause anaphylaxis during pregnancy, which has been associated with maternal and foetal death.

During labour and delivery, asthma medication should be used. In combination with hydration and adequate analgesia, medication may be enough to keep symptoms under control. Even acute exacerbation of asthma rarely requires caesarean delivery, because most women respond to aggressive medical management. Use of asthma medications can continue after delivery and during breastfeeding.

Women who are better educated about asthma management and how it relates to pregnancy often have an easier time controlling their symptoms. Pregnant asthmatic patients should be counselled to start rescue therapy at home if they experience symptoms of asthma flare-up, such as coughing, chest tightness, wheezing, shortness of breath, or laboured breathing. All women with asthma should be instructed to be attentive to foetal activity.

The successful management of asthma during pregnancy requires a cooperative approach between obstetricians and midwives, the physician, nurse specialists managing the asthma, and the woman herself. The aims and principles of treatment are the same as in the nonpregnant patient, and asthma should be treated as aggressively in pregnant women as in nonpregnant women. Pregnancy, because of the increased contact with health-care professionals, provides an ideal opportunity to optimise asthma management and, in many cases, to diagnose asthma for the first time. Home peak flow monitoring and personalised self-management plans are successful in the well-motivated pregnant asthmatic patient. The avoidance of asthma triggers is as important as in the nonpregnant patient.

The drug treatment of asthma in pregnancy is similar to the treatment of asthma in nonpregnant women, with a short-acting symptom reliever medication and long-term daily medication to address the underlying inflammation. However, it must be remembered that strong and repeated reassurance regarding the importance and safety of regular medication is needed to ensure compliance. All the drugs commonly used to treat asthma, including short- and long-acting β_2 agonists, inhaled corticosteroids, and methyl xanthines are safe in pregnancy. Fluticasone may be used for those requiring high doses of inhaled steroids.

ORAL CORTICOSTEROIDS

Because systemic corticosteroids have serious and well-known side effects when given frequently or in high doses for prolonged periods, women and their doctors are reluctant to use steroids in pregnancy. Most of this concern is misplaced, and steroids should be used to treat asthma in pregnancy in the same way and for the same reasons as outside pregnancy.

Prednisolone is metabolised by the placenta and very little (10 percent) active drug ever reaches the foetus. Several studies suggest no increased risk of abortion, stillbirth, congenital malformations, adverse foetal effects, or neonatal death attributable to treating the mother with steroids. There is a forty-six-year-old report of an increased incidence of cleft palate in the offspring of rabbits treated with cortisone early in gestation, and one recent retrospective study of 1184 cases of cleft lip suggested a possible association with oral corticosteroid treatment. Of the five affected pregnancies in the latter study, two were complicated by multiple congenital abnormalities, and in another case the mother was taking only replacement steroids for Addison's disease. Thus, only two pregnancies (no more than control) were complicated by isolated cleft lip in women taking therapeutic doses of corticosteroids. A larger case-control study of 20 830 cases of congenital abnormality revealed no association between the rate of different congenital abnormalities and corticosteroid treatment in the second and third months of gestation. There have been more recent concerns regarding possible deleterious effects of steroids later in gestation on foetal growth and lung and neuronal development and on hypertension. In addition, as discussed above, the association between asthma and preterm labour may in part be due to corticosteroid therapy, and this association is also described for other medical conditions treated with oral corticosteroids in pregnancy.

The maternal adverse effects from steroid therapy in pregnancy include increased risk of infections and reduced glucose tolerance and increase in gestational diabetes. The blood glucose should be checked regularly, and hyperglycaemia should be managed with insulin if necessary. The development of hyperglycaemia is not an indication to discontinue or decrease the dose of oral steroids, the requirement for which must be determined by the asthma. The rare but important psychiatric side effects of oral glucocorticoids should be remembered, and all women who have been started on steroids should be reviewed within one week.

An increased risk of pregnancy induced hypertension and preeclampsia has been reported in asthmatic women treated with oral corticosteroids. However, given the maternal and foetal consequences of severe asthma, the use of oral corticosteroids remains clinically indicated in pregnancy.

Thus, inhaled corticosteroids prevent exacerbations of asthma in pregnancy and are the prophylactic treatment of choice. The addition of systemic corticosteroids to control exacerbations of asthma is appropriate.

References

1-The American College of Obstetricians and Gynaecologists, Practice Bulletin #90. Asthma in pregnancy. February 2008, Obstetrics & Gynecology.

2-Nelson-Piercy, C. Asthma in pregnancy. Thorax, Volume 56, issue

Monochorionic Twin Gestation

OSCE station

Candidate Instructions

Mrs. S. has just had her booking scan in the foetal medicine department. The midwife in the day assessment unit asked her not to go home before you review the patient.

The scan report shows intrauterine twin gestation equivalent to eleven weeks with two amniotic sacs. There is a clear T sign at the membrane placental interface.

1) How you going to council the patient?

2) How is your diagnosis going to affect her antenatal care?

3) What complications, and how to avoid them, are to be discussed?

Examiner Instructions

Mrs. S. is thirty-eight years old with long history of subfertility. She had three previous unsuccessful IVFs. She managed to conceive in her fourth attempt. Her pregnancy so far has progressed in a satisfactory way. She is coming today for her booking scan, and her NT scan is already booked in a few days.

She is delighted with her pregnancy and looking forward to seeing her obstetrician in order to discuss the antenatal care plan. She has no special birth plans, though she prefers to have a normal delivery with a water birth.

Marking Sheet

1) How you going to council the patient?

Reassure   0 1

Monochorionic (MC) twins   0 1

Increased risk of complications   0 1

Be seen in a specialist consultant   0 1 2

Lead clinic

More intensive antenatal care   0 1

2) How is your diagnosis going to affect her antenatal care?

Detailed anamoly scan with cardiac screen   0 1 2

Serial growth scan (two to three weeks).   0 1

Report sudden increase in abdominal size or breathlessness.   01

Vaginal birth is appropriate in absence of complications.   01

Mode of delivery decision at thirty-six to thirty-seven weeks   0 1

3) What complications to be discussed ?

Twin–twin transfusion   0 1 2

Discordant foetal growth   0 1 2

Preeclampsia   0 1

Primary pulmonary hypertension (PPH)   0 1

Preterm birth   0 1

Discussion

This station tests the candidate's understanding of twins' gestation physiology, types, degree of risks, and complications associated with monochorionic diamniotic (MCDA) type. The diagram below show the different types of twins. Among them MCDA is the commonest type of monozygotic (identical) twins. While most obstetric complications are commoner in twins, twin–twin transfusion (TTTS) is one specific complication to MC twins, in which the twins have their circulations connected by placental blood vessels. The syndrome occurs in approximately 10 percent of monochorionic pregnancies and results from unequal blood exchange from one twin (donor) to the cotwin (recipient) through placental vascular anastomoses. Three types of placental anastomoses that connect intertwin circulation can be detected in all monochorionic placentas: arterio-arterial anastomoses, venovenous anastomoses, and arteriovenous anastomoses. The first type seems to have a protective role, because it balances blood shunting between the two foetuses. Conversely, arteriovenous capillary bed generates TTTS because of unbalanced flow from the donor to the recipient's circulation. Arteriovenous anastomoses from the recipient to the donor can also be present and compensate shunting from arteriovenous anastomoses from the donor to the recipient. However, when this compensation fails to balance intertwin blood shunting, TTTS develops. Because the vascular connections are responsible for hypovolaemia in the donor and hypervolaemia in the recipient, and because renal function is impaired in both twins, oligohydramnios develops in the donor's sac, and polyhydramnios develops in the recipient's sac. Therefore, the diagnosis of TTTS comprises sonographic detection of oligohydramnios (maximal vertical pocket ≤ 2 cm) and polyhydramnios (maximal vertical pocket ≥ 8 cm) in the donor and recipient sacs, respectively.

Foetal death of one twin places the surviving twin at increased risk of mortality and morbidity because of disseminated intravascular coagulation due to the passage of thromboplastic material from the dead foetus to the surviving foetus through placental vascular anatomizes.

The treatment of monochorionic pregnancies complicated with TTTS is based on the physiopathology described above. The following treatments have been described: amniodrainage, septostomy, laser photocoagulation of placental vascular anastomoses, and selective foeticide by umbilical cord occlusion.

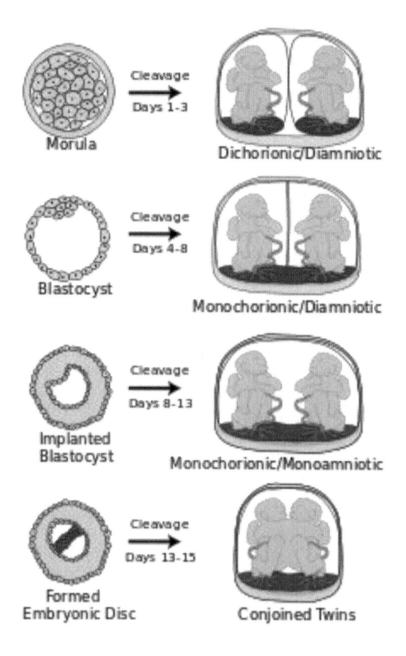

Figure 10: Types of Twin

References

1. Lewi, L.; Cannie, M; Blickstein, I; et al. Placental sharing, birth weight discordance, and vascular anastomoses in monochorionic diamniotic twin placentas. *Am. J. Obstet. Gynecol.* 197(6), 587.e1–587.e8 (2007).

2. Machin, G; Still, K; and Lalani, T. Correlations of placental vascular anatomy and clinical outcomes in 69 monochorionic twin pregnancies. *Am. J. Med. Genet.* 61(3), 229–236 (1996).

3. Guilherme, R; Patrier, S; Gubler, M. C.; Lemercier, D; Guimiot, F; and Dommergues, M. Very early twin-to-twin transfusion syndrome and discordant activation of the rennin–angiotensin system. *Placenta* 30(8), 731–734 (2009).

4. Quintero, R. A.; Morales, W. J.; Allen, M. H.; Bornick, P. W.; Johnson, P. K.; and Kruger, M. Staging of twin–twin transfusion syndrome. *J. Perinatol.* 19(8 Pt. 1), 550–555 (1999).

Sickle Cell Disease (SCD)

OSCE Station

Candidate Instructions

Mrs. K. is coming to see you in the preconception clinic. She immigrated from Tanzania a few years age as a teenager. She is now twenty-seven years old and planning to get pregnant soon. The only thing in her medical history is the diagnosis of sickle cell anaemia, for which she is a regular patient of the regional blood disorder clinic.

1) What are the important elements to discuss about her condition and pregnancy?

2) How you going to assess her?

3) What are the general aspects of her antenatal care?

Examiner Instructions

Mrs. K. is a case of SCD (Hb SS), which was diagnosed at the age of nineteen in one of UK's blood disorders centres. She had few episodes of sickling crisis in the last twenty-four months; the latest was just two months ago. She was admitted through accident and emergency (A&E) with extreme bone aches, for which she needed five days admission and few units of blood transfusion. On discharge her haemoglobin was 8.2 g/dl.

Her latest kidney and liver functions tests were within the acceptable range; however, previously she had a mild elevation of liver enzymes.

She was told that she is suffering from a heart valve condition that is unrelated to her SCD, and also her latest serum ferritin was 180 ng/ml.

Marking Sheet

1) What are the important elements to discuss about her condition and pregnancy?

Full history	0	1
Assess severity	0	1
Role of dehydration, cold	0	1
Risk of worsening anaemia	0	1
Risk of worsening crisis	0	1
risk of increased infection (UTI)	0	1
Increased risk of intrauterine growth restriction (IUGR)	0	1
Risk of induction of labour	0	1
Increased risk of CS	0	1
Chance baby is affected by SCD	0	1

2) How you going to assess her?

Assess for pulmonary hypertension	0	1
Cardiac scanning	0	1
Renal and liver function	0	1
Retinal screening	0	1
Iron overload	0	1

3) What are the general aspects of her antenatal care?

Multidisciplinary team	0	1
Haematologist check of end organ damage	0	1
Avoiding extreme temperatures, dehydration, and overexertion	0	1
Influenza vaccine	0	1
Partner checking	0	1

Discussion

The term SCD includes sickle cell anaemia (HbSS) and the heterozygous conditions of haemoglobin S and other clinically abnormal haemoglobins. These include combination with haemoglobin

C (giving Hb SC), combination with beta-thalassaemia (giving HbSB thalassaemia) and combination with haemoglobin D, E, or O-Arab. All of these genotypes will give a similar clinical phenotype of varying severity. Haemoglobin S combined with normal haemoglobin (A), known as sickle trait (AS), is asymptomatic, except for a possible increased risk of urinary tract infections and microscopic haematuria.

SCD is the most common inherited condition worldwide. About 300 000 children with SCD are born each year; two thirds of these births are in Africa. In the United Kingdom, it is estimated that there are 12 000–15 000 affected individuals, and over 300 infants born with SCD in the UK each year who are diagnosed as part of the neonatal screening programme.

Information that is particularly relevant for women planning to conceive includes the following:

Dehydration, cold, hypoxia, overexertion, and stress play a role in the frequency of sickle cell crises. Nausea and vomiting in pregnancy can result in dehydration and the precipitation of crises. Also the risk of worsening anaemia, the increased risk of crises and acute chest syndrome (ACS), and the risk of increased infection (especially UTI) during pregnancy. There is increased risk of

having a growth-restricted baby, which increases the likelihood of foetal distress, induction of labour, CS, and the chance of their baby being affected by SCD.

Women should be given H. influenza type B and the conjugated meningococcal C vaccine as a single dose if they have not received it as part of primary vaccination. The pneumococcal vaccine (Pneumovax®, Sanofi Pasteur MSD Limited, Maidenhead, UK) should be given every five years.

Women with SCD should be advised to receive the influenza and "swine flu" vaccine annually.

There is some evidence that the incidence of venous thromboembolism is increased among pregnant women with SCD. Thromboprophylaxis advice should be based on the RCOG Green-Top Guideline for women with additional risk factors. The use of graduated compression stockings of appropriate strength is recommended in pregnancy for women considered to be at risk of venous thromboembolism, as discussed in the RCOG Green-Top Guideline on thromboprophylaxis.

Painful crisis is the most frequent complication of SCD during pregnancy, with between 27 and 50 percent of women having a painful crisis during pregnancy, and it is the most frequent cause of hospital admission. Avoidance of precipitants such as a cold environment, excessive exercise, dehydration, and stress is important. Mild pain may be managed in the community with rest, oral fluids, and paracetamol or weak opioids. NSAIDs should be used only between twelve and twenty-eight weeks of gestation.

Acute anaemia in women with SCD may be attributable to *Erythrovirus* infection. Infection with *Erythrovirus* in SCD causes a red-cell maturation arrest and an aplastic crisis characterised by a reticulocytopenia. Therefore, a reticulocyte count should be requested in any woman presenting with an acute anaemia and, if low, may indicate infection with *Erythrovirus*. Treatment is with blood transfusion, and the woman must be isolated. With

Erythrovirus infection there is the added risk of vertical transmission to the foetus, which can result in hydrops foetalis, hence a review by a foetal medicine specialist is needed.

Thromboembolism (VTE)

OSCE Station

Candidate Instructions

Mrs. F. is thirty-nine years old, pregnant with her third baby at thirty-two weeks. Midwife has asked her to go to the day assessment unit (DAU) because of severe right upper thigh pain. On arrival to the DAU you were asked to see her.

1) How you going to assess her?

2) What is the most likely diagnosis, and how you going to confirm it?

3) What further management does she need?

Examiner Instructions

Mrs. F. is pregnant with her third baby, thirty-two weeks' gestation; her pregnancy has been uneventful so far. The first baby was delivered by emergency CS due to delayed second stage and malposition; second baby was delivered by elective CS. In this pregnancy she has noticed gradual swelling of her right upper thigh, which was getting worse day by day, in addition to increasing pain and difficulty in walking. In fact, most of her right leg is swollen now, with redness and soreness in the region of femoral triangle.

There is no personal history of thrombosis; however, there is a family history of DVT in both her mum and sister. Mother developed DVT spontaneously, while her sister had it following hysterectomy. She does not smoke or drink; her BMI is 29 kg/m2.

Marking Sheet

1) How you going to assess her?

History of complaint	0	1
Past personal history	0	1
Past family history	0	1
General examination	0	1
Local examination	0	1
Foetal assessment		

2) What is the most likely diagnosis, and how you going to confirm it?

DVT	0	1	2
Compression duplex US	0	1	2
Clotting profile	0	1	2
FBC, LFT, U&E	0	1	2

Thrombophilia screen   0   1   2

3) What further management does she need?

Start LMW heparin before diagnosis and afterward   0   1

Leg elevation   0   1

Graduated stock compression   0   1

Heparin for whole pregnancy, and six weeks postnatal   0   1

Postnatal clinic review   0   1

Discussion

Routine thromboprophylaxis is currently recommended only for
pregnant women considered at high risk for venous thromboembolism (VTE) on the basis of certain factors such as a previous
VTE, but disagreement and inconsistency prevail regarding the
characteristics that put women at higher risk for development of
a first VTE during pregnancy or postpartum. To identify women
who would benefit most from thromboprophylaxis, it is essential to
determine the absolute risk (AR) for VTE in women during pregnancy and how potential risk factors actually affect this risk.

VTE remains the main direct cause of maternal death in the UK,
and many reports of *Confidential Enquiries into Maternal Deaths*
have highlighted failures in obtaining objective diagnoses and
employing adequate treatment. The subjective, clinical assessment of deep venous thrombosis (DVT) and pulmonary throm

boembolism (PTE) is particularly unreliable in pregnancy, and a minority of women with clinically suspected VTE have the diagnosis confirmed when objective testing is employed. However, VTE is up to ten times more common in pregnant women than in nonpregnant women of the same age and can occur at any stage of pregnancy, but the puerperium is the time of highest risk. The symptoms and signs of VTE include leg pain and swelling (usually unilateral), lower abdominal pain, low-grade pyrexia, dyspnoea, chest pain, haemoptysis, and collapse.

Compression duplex ultrasound is the primary diagnostic test for DVT. If ultrasound confirms the diagnosis of DVT, anticoagulant treatment should be continued. If ultrasound is negative, and a high level of clinical suspicion exists, the woman should remain anticoagulated and ultrasound repeated in one week or an alternative diagnostic test employed. If repeat testing is negative, anticoagulant treatment should be discontinued.

When iliac vein thrombosis is suspected (back pain and swelling of the entire limb), magnetic resonance venography or conventional contrast venography may be considered.

Performing a thrombophilia screen prior to therapy is controversial, and it is therefore not routinely recommended. This is because the results of a thrombophilia screen will not influence immediate management of acute VTE, but it can provide information that can influence the duration and intensity of anticoagulation.

If a thrombophilia screen is performed, it is important to be aware of the effects of pregnancy and thrombus on the results of a thrombophilia screen. For example, protein S levels fall in normal pregnancy, making it extremely difficult to make a diagnosis of protein S deficiency during pregnancy. Activated protein C (APC) resistance is found in around 40 percent of pregnancies, owing to the physiological changes in the coagulation system. Antithrombin may be reduced when extensive thrombus is present.

Meta-analyses of randomised controlled trials indicate that low molecular weight heparins (LMWHs) are more effective, are associated with a lower risk of haemorrhagic complications, and are associated with lower mortality than unfractionated heparin in the initial treatment of DVT in nonpregnant women.

Pain and swelling in the affected leg are debilitating symptoms of DVT. Short-term studies in patients with proximal DVT showed that pain and swelling improved faster in mobile patients wearing compression hosiery than in those resting in bed without any compression. This approach can also prevent the development of post-thrombotic syndrome. Below-knee compression socks are acceptable for patients without thigh or knee swelling.

Studies in the nonpregnant have shown that early mobilisation with compression therapy does not increase the likelihood of developing PTE. Thus, there is no requirement for bed rest in a stable patient on anticoagulant treatment with acute DVT.

OSCE Station

Preterm Labour

Candidate Instructions

The patient you about to see has just been admitted to your maternity unit. The midwife is concerned about her, and no other doctor is available to see her at present.

You have fifteen minutes to take a history; you should obtain information relevant to her current pregnancy, determine the reason for her admission, and formulate a management plan.

You will be awarded marks for your ability to take a history, make a diagnosis, and formulate management plan.

Role-player Instructions

You have a disinterested attitude.

You are eighteen years old, this is your second pregnancy, and you are now twenty-nine weeks.

It is an unplanned pregnancy from a casual relationship. Your previous pregnancy was terminated at eight weeks, as you were then only fifteen and still at school. You booked at the maternity hospital at sixteen weeks. All bloods were normal. You have shared care with your GP.

Ultrasound at eighteen weeks showed a normally grown foetus equivalent to your dates. The scan noted a choroid plexus cyst. You were seen by the consultant and reassured. Rescan at twenty-four weeks confirmed the disappearance of the cyst.

The day before admission, you felt generally unwell with cramp abdominal pains.

Several hours before admission, you developed abdominal pains that were intermittent and are now lasting about thirty seconds with two to three minutes in between. You have also had some vaginal discharge that is slimy with some blood staining.

Personal: single, unemployed, live at home with parents and three brothers and two sisters. You are the eldest.

Family: mother is nonidentical twin.

Drugs: occasional Ecstasy, but not since you knew about pregnancy; inhaler and asthma

You have to ask the candidate what is the cause of pain.

Examiner's Instructions

This is an unplanned teenage pregnancy complicated by premature labour at twenty-nine weeks' gestation. The role of the candidate is to take a full history. The candidate must evaluate the condition of the patient, and full examination and speculum examination and swabs must be taken. Adequate sedation must be given to control the pain and tocolytic agent should be initiated. Evaluate ultrasound of the baby, placenta, and liquor volume. Two doses of steroid must be given to achieve lung maturity.

The candidate should provide a good explanation to the patient and keep good communication skills and allow patient to ask questions.

Marking Sheet

1- Introduction

   Nonmedical language

   Eye contact

   Listen to patient

   Allow questions   0 1 2 3 4 5

2- Past history

   Obstetric

   Social

   Drugs

   Family

   Medical   0 1 2 3 4 5

3- Provisional diagnosis

Preterm labour

Investigate cause

Infection   0   1   2   3   4   5

4- Treatment plan

Admit

Speculum examination

Stop contractions

Steroids   0   1   2   3   4   5

Discussion

Preterm birth remains the leading public health problem in obstetrics. A recent analysis of neonatal mortality (death at less than twenty days) in the United States between 1989 and 2001 revealed that extremely preterm delivery (less than twenty-eight weeks' gestation) accounted for 49 to 58 percent of these deaths, and preterm delivery (less than thirty-seven weeks) accounted for 70 percent of neonatal deaths. In addition to being at risk for neonatal death, preterm infants are at increased risk for long-term neurologic and developmental morbidity.

Despite major clinical research efforts aimed at reducing the incidence of preterm births, the preterm birth rate reached its highest level in two decades: 11.9 percent in 2001. Similarly, the preterm birth rate has risen 27 percent since 1981. Much of this increase may be accounted for by the increase in multiple gestations brought about by assisted reproductive technology. However, the preterm birth rate among singletons has also risen during this time period.

Evidence regarding efficacy of interventions to prevent preterm birth has been disappointing. Most studies have failed to demonstrate any reduction in preterm births with such interventions (e.g., home uterine activity monitoring, administration of tocolytics, and intensive and frequent contact with health-care providers). Recently progesterone has shown some promise in the prevention of preterm birth among women with prior preterm births. Whether this intervention will prove effective in other populations, such as women with multiple gestations, remains to be seen.

Markers for predicting preterm birth, such as foetal fibronectin and transvaginal cervical length, may provide a means of differentiating between those women truly at risk for preterm birth and those destined to deliver at term.

Cervical length measurement has traditionally been used to assess high-risk patients for cervical insufficiency, as manifested by some degree of cervical shortening, plus/minus funnelling of the membranes into the internal os.

Numerous observational studies have been performed assessing the test characteristics of cervical length assessment for prediction of spontaneous preterm birth.

To date, the most extensively studied marker of preterm birth is foetal fibronectin. Foetal fibronectin is a glycoprotein found in high concentrations in the amniotic fluid and in the interface between the decidua and the trophoblast cells. Although normally found in the cervical and vaginal secretions before sixteen to twenty weeks gestation, its presence in the cervicovaginal secretion after twenty weeks' gestation is abnormal, except as a marker of preterm labour. This elevation of foetal fibronectin levels is thought to reflect mechanical or inflammatory damage to the membranes or placenta. The foetal fibronectin cutoff for a positive test is ≥ 50 ng/mL.

Because of the predictive ability of cervical length measurements at eighteen to twenty-four weeks' gestation among asymptomatic women, transvaginal cervical length measurement has been used to identify a group of women who might benefit from cervical cerclage. To date, there have been three randomized controlled trials evaluating the therapeutic effectiveness of cervical cerclage among asymptomatic women with short cervices diagnosed by ultrasound. Disappointingly, two of these studies (one of these a large multicenter effort) showed no benefit to cervical cerclage.

OSCE Station

No Foetal Movements

Candidate Information

Mrs. P. Edward is a twenty-six-year-old primigravida who is forty-one weeks pregnant. She is admitted to labour ward with a history of no foetal movements for forty-eight hours. A senior midwife has been unable to pick up the foetal heartbeat with the CTG.

You have been asked to see her.

Role-Player Information

You are an anxious twenty-six-year-old bank clerk in your second pregnancy. You have previously had a miscarriage at ten weeks' gestation. You are now forty-one weeks pregnant, and for the past two days you have not felt any foetal movements. There is no history of abdominal pain or vaginal bleeding. However, you have felt a little off-colour over the past few days.

When you contacted your community midwife, she came to see you and was unable to hear the baby's heart with the Doppler. She advised you to go straight to hospital.

You are very anxious and frightened. Husband is on his way from work. When you know the diagnosis you are upset and angry. You are over your expected date of delivery and had wanted to be induced early on but had been told by your midwife that this is not possible till forty-two weeks.

A hospital midwife has been unable to detect the baby's heartbeat with a CTG.

The candidate is expected to take a history from you and ask to examine your abdomen. The candidate should then explain the following points to you. If the candidate does not cover these points, then you should ask direct questions regarding the following:

1) The baby may have died, and in order to confirm, an ultrasound scan is needed. (This scan will confirm death and reveal an estimated foetal weight of 2.8 kg and reduced liquor).

2) Candidate will explain result of scan in a clear and sympathetic manner. He or she should ask if anyone is with you.

3) The possible cause is a placental insufficiency, but this needs to be confirmed.

You should ask that whether being overdue has contributed to foetal death. You should also ask why you were not induced when you requested that.

4) The candidate should explain why you were not induced before forty-one weeks.

5) The candidate should explain that you need to be delivered and that this does not need to be done today. He or she should explain that you might go into labour on your own, but you should not be left for days because of risk to you. They should advise that this delivery is to be carried out within the next seventy-two hours.

6) Method of induction of labour.

7) They should advise you to have postmortem for the baby to find out the cause of death.

8) Several tests will need to be carried out (blood test for diabetes, clotting, swabs for infection, liver and renal function, placenta for histology, etc.).

9) Photos, footprints, funeral arrangement, imam or priest.

10) Stillbirth support group/SANDS.

Examiner Instruction

P. E. is twenty-seven years old in her first pregnancy; so far her pregnancy was uneventful, but over the last twenty-four hours, she did not feel the foetal movement. She is forty-one weeks' gestation, and her induction of labour day is next week. She was worried about the baby being overdue and felt her tummy is a bit small and asked the midwife if she can be induced.

Today she went to see her community midwife about lack of baby's movements. The midwife confirmed that she cannot hear foetal heart and referred her to local labour ward. Midwife on labour ward could not hear the foetal heart and called the registrar on call. The registrar should examine the abdomen and confirm foetal demise with scan. He or she should then explain the scan finding and plan of action with regard to delivery and investigation.

Foetal scan: intrauterine foetal death, estimated foetal weight (EFW) is 2.8 kg, reduced liquor.

Result to be given to the candidate if he/she asked for ultrasound.

Marking Sheet

1- Communication

   Introduction.

   Establish rapport.

   Ask if she is alone/anybody with her.

   Find out how she is feeling.

   Use plain and simple language.

   Allow her to ask questions.

   Do not give reason for foetal death.

   Do not put blame on anyone.

   Give clear plan of action.

   Provide reassurance   0 1 2 3 4 5 6 7 8 9 10

2- Knowledge

   Need for ultrasound and findings/small baby with reduced liquor

   Likely cause of death but not definitive

Possible other causes

Reason for induction at forty-two weeks   0 1 2 3 4 5

C) Management

Arrangement for induction (when?)

Method of delivery

Investigations

Postmortem/Full; limited; if declined, why

Baby funeral arrangement/photos, footprint (should offer these after delivery)

Support groups/SANDS   0 1 2 3 4 5

Discussion

Sudden foetal death is one of the most tragic events parents can be subjected to. Most of the time, the tragedy happens in the least expected manner, and therefore the shock would be most profound. The natural reaction of any parent, beside the extreme sadness, is the burning desire to know why it happened. Could it have been prevented? Who should be blamed for that?

The caregiver must show great sympathy and a gentle approach to any initial questions, taking great care not to give a definite answer before all investigations are completed. The cause of foetal death should be determined whenever possible. Only then can the likelihood of a recurrence and the possibility of prevention be ascertained.

Maternal and family history should be obtained by the attending obstetrician, followed by careful examination of the mother and ultrasound examination of the baby in search for the cause of death.

Carefully examine the baby and placenta after birth, looking for any obvious abnormalities that can give explanation to what happened. Parent consent should be obtained for postmortem examination after full explanation of the likely benefit obtained from such procedure.

Induction of labour must be planned; parents should be given the choice about the timing of induction. Early induction has many advantages, including early healing, and postmortem will be yielding more useful information before establishment of autolysis. Psychosocial support is very important, to be started immediately, to expedite the healing process.

There is a long list of investigations needed to aid in finding the cause of this tragedy, including screening for coagulopathy, infection screening, antibodies testing, and sometimes karyotyping of parents.

During induction of labour, one-to-one care, adequate analgesia, and undisturbed environment should be available for the couple in all labour wards. Maternity departments nowadays offer psychological support via specialist midwife and counsellor to facilitate the grieving process and speed up the healing and maintain communications and feedback. The parents can contact local and national support groups such as SAND for further advice and support. The parent should be encouraged to hold the baby and keep the baby in the room with them to create bonding and establish the parenthood feeling. Neonatal footprint, handprints, and photographs should be obtained, and every effort should be taken to encourage the parents to name the baby.

Obstetrics OSCE Station

Postnatal Collapse

Candidate Instruction

A thirty-nine-year-old Nigerian woman, P4 (all SVD 1.5–4 hours), was admitted for induction of labour at thirty-eight weeks' gestation. She has had normal antenatal care so far. Her blood investigations revealed Hb AS (SS trait), O Pos, BMI 30. She is a nonsmoker and does not drink alcohol. She is known to have gestational diabetes and is on metformin. Foetal growth revealed large for gestational age (LFD) baby; FBC showed the following:

Hb	107 g/l
MCV	83
HCT	31.2
WBC	5.1
Plt	86

She had 1 mg of prostaglandin at 9.44 hours and 1 mg at 17.28 hours, followed by artificial rupture of membranes at 19.38 hours; liquor was meconium-stained.

CTG remained normal throughout. During labour, midwife noticed tachypnoea thought to be labour-pain-related.

1- Assess the information above

2- State your action

Second part

Baby and placenta delivered at 21.53 hours, foetal weight was 4 100 g, and blood loss of 250 ml; Syntometrin given at 21.54 hours. She became profoundly short of breath; however, chest examinations revealed no wheeze.

General observations at 22.10 hours showed the following:

Respiratory rate (RR)	44/m
O2 saturations	77% in air
Heart rate (HR)	86 beats/m
BP	154/84 mmhg
Temperature	36.9 C

1-Put in an immediate plan of management.

2-What other investigation would you like to order?

3-What other signs and symptoms would you enquire about?

Third Part

Blood Results Before and After Delivery

Before delivery

Hb 107, MCV 83, HCT 31.2, WCC 5.1, Plt 86, EBL 200 ml, approx. 250ml IV fluid given.

Repeated same day after delivery

Hb 137, MCV 83.2, HCT 39.1, WCC 7.4, Plt 110

UE / LFT / CRP / coagulation profile—all were normal.

1-What is your differential diagnosis?

2-What is the priority management?

Fourth Part

The following imaging were requested and reported as follows:

19/11/13 chest X-ray (CXR)—diffuse parahilar haziness consistent with pulmonary oedema/acute respiratory distress syndrome (ARDS)?

19/11/13 CT pulmonary angiogram (CTPA)—Bilateral dependant, and some degree of perihilar lung consolidations are noted? Pulmonary oedema? ARDS?

1- Your immediate action

2- Would you plan further investigations or intervention?

Examiner's Notes

This pregnant lady reported during her antenatal booking that she had rheumatic fever as a child; however, no antenatal complication was reported. Her induction of labour was carried out by PGE2 and was straightforward. The in-charge midwife noticed tachypnea and low saturation, which was immediately treated with high O2 flow with face mask after delivery.

The immediate working provisional diagnosis is of acute cardiomyopathy or amniotic fluid embolism.

Blood picture and imaging indicated acute respiratory condition with low platelet count, low O2 saturation, and high haematocrit.

The working diagnosis was ARDS; this will require multidisciplinary approach and early involvement of medical team and ITU team in addition to imaging department. Therefore it was decided to transfer this patient to ITU.

ITU admission for four days—intubated, daily CXR—successfully weaned, and patient recovered completely and transferred back to labour HDU.

Sputum for adenovirus, *Coxiellaci burnetii*, *Chlamydia*, influenza A, influenza B, *Mycoplasma pneumoniae*, parainfluenza, and respiratory syncytial virus were all *negative*.

Legionella antigen was *not* detected, and MSU was negative.

Cardiology opinion was sought and confirmed the diagnosis of *postpartum heart failure*; echo test showed mild left ventricle (LV) hypertrophy and moderate mitral stenosis. She was started on bisoprolol and frusemide.

Marking Sheet

1- Candidate should identify the severity of the condition, which may be precipitated by Syntometrine injection. 0 1 2 3

2- Blood result needs to be identified to make a plan of management. 0 1 2 3

3- Further investigation would be arterial blood and imaging investigation. 0 1 2 3

4- Request a multidisplinary approach. 0 1 2 3

5- Interpret the CXR and CTPA. 0 1 2 3 4

6- Obtain a differential diagnosis of ARDS cardiomyopathy and amniotic fluid embolism. 0 1 2 3 4

Discussion

This is an acute respiratory condition characterised by low O2 saturation and low platelets and high haematocrit; in addition the imaging indicated some lungs features. Cardiac echo indicated mitral valve disease due to previous rheumatic fever.

The lung syndrome is inflammation of lung parenchyma, leading to impaired gas exchange with a systemic release of inflammatory mediators, causing inflammation, hypoxia, and multiple organ failure. This syndrome is associated with 90 percent death rate in untreated patients.

Signs and symptoms of respiratory failure cannot be explained by heart failure, volume overload, pleural effusion, pneumothorax, nodules, or airway obstruction.

CXR showed bilateral infiltrates sparing costophrenic angles. Sepsis in this case is unlikely, given the patient's immediate history. This picture can be explained by circulation overload by multiple blood transfusions. Also the picture can be explained by aspiration of gastric contents with or without drug overdose. Other possibilities can be included in the differential diagnosis, such as pancreatitis, pneumonia, and shock.

Amniotic Fluid Embolism

Acute and extensive amniotic fluid embolism (AFE sometimes do not have anything to do with lung injury. Treat first, then retrospectively look for causes. AFE is the fifth most common cause of perinatal mortality (1.8 cases per 100 000 maternities in UK).

AFE is associated with induction of labour and multiple pregnancies.

The main symptoms are bleeding diathesis, respiratory distress and cyanosis, hypotension, seizures, and collapse. Other symptoms are chest pain or bronchospasm.

CXR showed pulmonary oedema / ARDS, right atrial enlargement, and a prominent pulmonary artery.

ECG and arterial blood gases are unhelpful in diagnosis.

Postmortem will reveal foetal squamous cells and lanugo hair in the maternal pulmonary circulation.

The primary management strategy is immediate transfer to ITU and assisted ventilation.

Obstetrics Preparatory OSCE Station

Medicolegal Case

Candidate Instruction

This is a preparatory station; you have fifteen minutes to read and utilise your opinion about the claim, and you will then move to the the next station, where you will meet a consultant who will ask you questions about the claim and how to defend your management.

You are special registrar (SpR) year three in obstetrics and gynaecology; your consultant asks you to read the following management of this patient and write a report about the claim that was sent by her husband and claimed poor management on the labour ward. You were on duty that day when she was on the labour ward, and you are among other doctors and midwives looking after her.

- Thirty-five years Po+1 spontaneous pregnancy; she was booked for consultant-led care at 16/40. She is a known Jehovah's Witness and declared at booking that she would not accept blood and some blood products. Her BMI is 18, and her booking observation is as follows:

- Booking BP 120/76

- Rhesus—negative

- No significant medical /surgical past history

- Red dye foods allergy

- Would accept clotting factors or albumin but no red cells.

The patient was given general advice, including diet to maintain Hb level and avoid anaemia.

- Anti-D at 28 weeks was discussed.

- Declined Anti-D (partner Rh+ve).

- Hb 10 gms/dl and has been prescribed ferrous sulphate oral tablets, 200 mg twice daily, from 31+ weeks.

She was referred to consultant antenatal clinic for further discussion.

- Accepted Anti-D at 35+/40 and was administered.

She had private vaginal swab, which confirmed GBS positive.

- Hb at 37/40 was 11.5 gms/dl

- At 40/40, patient self referred for per vaginal fluid loss

  - Clinical examination did not confirm ruptured membranes on speculum inspection.

She was admitted for observation, and (PAD) test did not confirm passage of liquor.

  - Ultrasound scan at 40/40 showed normal liquor volume, normal amniotic fluid index and normal growth.

She was discharged home.

She was admitted at term +2 with spontaneous labour with regular uterine contractions, to antenatal ward at 2.40 hours.

- Transferred to LW due to concerns of midwife with foetal heart.

Vaginal examination revealed fully effaced and 4-cm-dilated cervix and absent membranes, and no liquor was seen.

8:30 a.m.

- CTG normal

- Plan active third-stage management

- Review by consultant on call at 9:45 a.m.

Inadequate uterine contractions were discovered, and it was decided to start her on Syntocinon augmentation, and the plan will be as follows:

- Vaginal examination in four hours from Syntocinon augmentation

- Active third-stage management

Patient was reviewed by the on-call registrar at 10.45 for the following:

- Prolonged bradycardia

- Vaginal examination showed cervix 6–7 cm dilated.

- Normal CTG; revert to normal after seven minutes.

- For foetal blood sampling (FBS), if further concerns with CTG

She was reviewed again by registrar on call at 15.20 hours

- Pathological CTG

    - For FBS, which was carried out and found the following:

    - PHvenous, 7.359; arterial, 7.306

    - Base excess (BE) -3.7   -2.5

    - Plan for STAN monitoring

- On STAN

Vaginal examination at 1630 hours showed the following:

    - Cervix fully dilated

    - Cephalic presentation: left occipitotransverse (LOT), vertex at spines

    - Significant ST events

- 1745 hours—Discussed with consultant on call

- Agreed for trial of instrumental delivery in theatre; if failed, the patient should be delivered by lower segment CS.

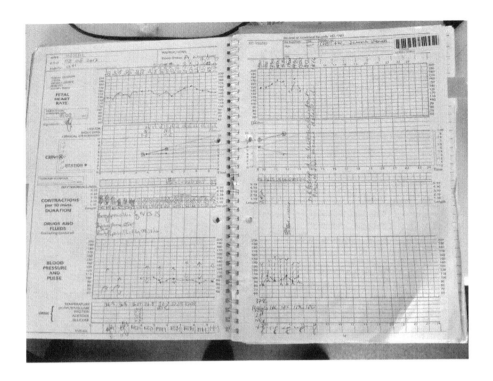

Figure: Partograme of the patient in this case

In Theatre

- Examination under anaesthesia (EUA) to check presentation and position; it was decided to apply the following:

- Ventouse vaginal delivery

  - Vertix rotated to right occipital anterior (ROA)

  - Cup pop off after two pulls

- Decision for midcavity forceps delivery, Neville Barnes C (NB) was applied, right lateral episiotomy was given, and the baby was delivered with two pulls.

- Episiotomy and lateral vaginal wall lacerations were sutured in theatre.

- 1 000 mls estimated blood loss.

Postrepair analgesia, hygiene, and care was discussed.

She was referred to A&E fifteen days postdelivery, as she was presented with heavy vaginal bleeding.

She was commenced on antibiotics, and a pelvic US was ordered to rule out retained products on conceptions (RPOCs).

She attended again eighteen days postdelivery and reviewed by gynaecology SHO. She was complaining of incontinence of bowel and bladder.

- Flatus incontinence

- O/E episiotomy healed well

- mild puckering at fourchette

  - Unable to control flatus at the time of examination

- Discussed with registrar on call, who got in touch with consultant on call; it was decided to give a perineal clinic referral.

Obstetric OSCE Station

Medicolegal Case

Examiner Instruction

Partner's Letter 10 Nov 2011

I am writing to complain about my wife's treatment when she had our first child on 10/06/12. I feel that many things should have been done before and during her labour that could have alleviated a lot of the stress that she has had and could have prevented the complications that we still trying to sort out.

1-She has a small birth canal, which made it hard for her to give birth. Therefore she should have been given caesarean section.

2-The birth itself was very traumatic on my wife; she was advised by midwife to stay at home, because she was not in labour, and on admission later, the baby's heart rate dropped dangerously, causing stress to the baby.

3-She was told by one staff when we requested caesarean section, "So you want to die" because we are Jehovah's Witnesses and refuse blood.

4-We were told that the cord was around the neck of the baby, leading to dropping of the baby's heart rate.

5-My wife was left to continue to go through agonising contractions, and my little baby was in distress, and every time a contraction happened, his heartbeat dropped, and still they refused to give my wife caesarean section, because we refused blood.

6-They left her to push for a long time and nothing happening.

7-They failed to deliver the baby with ventouse because the ventouse slipped off and she had to have forceps delivery. This clearly indicates that they put her under severe stress and denied her caesarean section.

8-She is still suffering from pain and discomfort down below and having problems with bladder and bowel control nearly six months later and has to have urodynamics and bowel scan.

9-She was referred to perineal clinic and was investigated but still could not control her bowel. For this referral we had to wait for nearly five months.

10-She has endured stress and anxiety caused by the whole experience, which has resulted in her suffering from postnatal depression.

11-She was referred for physiotherapy but with no benefit.

Solicitor's Letter 02 Sept. 2012

Re: Clinical Negligence Claim

Dear Sir:

We have been instructed by Mrs. N. G. in connection with an investigation into an allegation of negligence made against your trust, and relating to care afforded to her prior to and during the birth of her first child on 10/06/12.

In order to succeed in a clinical negligence claim, the claimant must be able to show the following:

1-That the defendant had a duty of care towards her.

2-That there was a breach of that duty of care.

3-There must have been foreseeable consequences, which were not too remote, and we consider, based upon evidence to date, that our client will be able to succeed in this respect; however, until we have fully investigated Mrs. N. G.'s treatment and dealt with the issue of liability, causation, condition, and prognosis, we are unable to quantify the value of this claim.

4-We are therefore requesting copy of her notes.

Marking Sheet

1- The likely nature of the claim   0 1

2- What is the ground of the claim   0 1

3- Any action taken by the hospital to answer the point mentioned by her husband in his letter to the trust   0 1

4- Solicitor is requesting the following:

     A. Photocopies of the notes   0 1

     B. Copies of computerised records   0 1

     C. Copies of baby's heart records   0 1

     D. Copies of X-rays, scans, and all tests   0 1

5- Caesarean section was indicated:

Small pelvis   0 1 2

Foetal heart dropping   0 1 2

She was told cannot have caesarean section, because she was refusing blood.   0 1

She was pushing for a long time.   0 1

Should not have had ventouse, as it was slipped on pulling. 0 1 2

6- Bladder and bowel trauma:

Waited five months before seen in the perineal clinic.   0 1

Did not benefit from the perineal clinic referral.   0 1

Did not benefit from physiotherapy.   0 1

7- Hospital failed their duty of care.   0 1 2 3

Discussion

In English tort law, an individual may owe a duty of care to another, to ensure that they do not suffer any unreasonable harm or loss. If such a duty is found to be breached, a legal liability is imposed upon the defender to compensate the victim for any losses they incur.

The first element of negligence is the legal duty of care. This concerns the relationship between the defendant (hospital and staff) and the claimant (patient), which must be such that there is an obligation upon the defendant to take proper care to avoid causing injury to the plaintiff (patient)in all the circumstances of the case. There are two ways in which a duty of care may be established:

1. The defendant and claimant are within one of the recognised relationships where a duty of care is established by precedent; or

2. outside these relationships, according to the principles developed by case law.

The principles delineated in *Caparo v. Dickman* specify a tripartite test:

1. Was the harm reasonably foreseeable?

2. Was there a requisite degree of proximity between the claimant and the defendant?

3. Is it fair, just, and reasonable to impose a duty of care—are there precluding public policy concerns?

There are a number of distinct and recognisable situations in which the courts recognise the existence of a duty of care. Examples include

- one road-user to another,

- employer to employee,

- manufacturer to consumer,

- doctor to patient, and

- solicitor to client.

Patient is entitled to copies of her notes, scans, and investigations and any foetal and maternal computerized recording; this can be requested by the patient and/or the solicitor.

There was no indication that this patient should be delivered by cae- sarean section; there is no evidence of cephalopelvic disproportion, and foetal heart rate deceleration was fully investigated, and foetal pH and base excess did not indicate the baby was in distress.

The use of vacuum extraction delivery is to rotate the foetal head to occipital anterior (OA) from LOT, and delivery can be achieved with ventouse or forceps.

Bladder and bowel dysfunction is not unusual after operative or even normal delivery. In this case there is no severe perineal trauma apart from uncomplicated episiotomy.

The dysfunction was investigated fully with urodynamic study, and rectal scan did not reveal any external or internal rectal sphincter injury.

Jehovah's Witnesses who refused blood and blood products should have signed and witnessed Advance Directive, and the policy should be noted and discussed during antenatal visits, and the anaesthetist must be informed, and in most of the cases an appointment is made to see the patient and discuss her request of no blood and blood products. The anaesthetist should inform the patient of availability of cell saver arrangement to collect the patient's own blood and reinfuse it to the patient.

Obstetrics OSCE Station

Mental Diseases

Candidate Instructions

While you were reviewing GP letters, you found this one:

Dear Doctor,

I would like you to see Mrs. Z. in your booking clinic. She is pregnant with her first baby at eight weeks' gestation. The main reason of referral is her long history of mental disorder. She was diagnosed with bipolar disorder six years back and had several treatments. Can you arrange to see her as soon as possible? Thanks!

1) What is your plan for her booking visit?

2) What is your plan for her antenatal care throughout pregnancy?

3) What is your care plan for labour and postnatal period?

Examiner Instructions

Mrs. Z. is twenty-one years old, para zero; at the age of fifteen, she was diagnosed with severe depression, for which she was started on antidepressant for six months. The diagnosis was then reviewed, and she was given the new label of mania depression. Her medications subsequently changed. After this diagnosis she had attempted her first suicide (medication overdose), for which she needed inpatient treatment for several weeks in a special institution for mental disease. She was discharged to the community afterward and was reviewed as an outpatient, till she changed her address and was lost to the follow-up. Three years ago she was admitted through A&E department with second attempt of overdose. This last attempt was worse than the first one; and this time she needed to stay in the ITU for three weeks. She was transferred again after recovery to another mental hospital and made a good recovery. Over the last eighteen months, she is back in the community, on regular medications for her condition, and she fully understands that if she abandons her treatment or follow-up she would stand the risk of being admitted to a mental institution with low chance of being released to the community.

Marking Sheet

1) What is your plan for her booking visit?

You have to uncover the following:

History of mental disorder   0 1

History of previous treatment and inpatient stay   0 1

Family history of mental disorder 0 1

Current treatment with antipsychotic 01

History of domestic violence 01 2

History of self-harm 0 1

History of sexual abuse/assault 0 1

Referral to psychiatric unit for those with risk factors 01 2

2) What is your plan for her antenatal care throughout pregnancy?

Special protocol to deal with such cases. 0 1

Screening questions about depression in each visit. 01 2

Drugs prescribed only if necessary. 01

Self-help strategies should be tried first. 012

Balance out risk of medication v. nontreatment. 012

Referral to specialist centres for severe cases. 0 1

Alcohol or drug abuse needs referral to drug centres. 01

3) What is your care plan for labour and postnatal period?

Agreed care plan. 01 2

One-to-one care. 012

Clear advice about antipsychotic medications in labour. 01

All procedures should be consented as per RCOG guidelines. 0 1

- Postnatal care plan by the team should be in place. 01

- Infants of mothers on medications should be observed. 0 1

- Share info on high-risk patients with GP, and mental team. 0 1

- Change in mental state needs urgent liaison with mental team. 0 1

Discussion

The issue of mental health in pregnancy is a very important one. While many patients enjoy a healthy mental status throughout pregnancy and puerperium, there are others who develop mental disease for the first time during pregnancy or, more commonly, postnatally. There are also many more who already had a background of mental diseases in the past, which make them more susceptible for it in pregnancy or puerperium.

The main task of any obstetrician is to uncover all risk factors early on in pregnancy and specifically at the booking visit. While depression and anxiety are the most common mental disorders that can be encountered, there are many other more serious conditions that can inflict great harm to both mother and baby (e.g., bipolar disease, schizophrenia, and various types of phobia).

Most patients with mental problems have this deep-rooted fear that their medications could harm their babies and therefore they should stop them before pregnancy. Many doctors also believe that the side effects of most antipsychotics cannot justify using them in the early stages of pregnancy. If the mental condition is one that can result in serious harm to patient if medications were to be discontinued, then the balance of risks is in favour of continuing the medications in pregnancy, regardless of the perceived risk of side effects.

Obstetrics OSCE Station

Ovarian Cyst during Pregnancy

Candidate Instruction

You are about to see Mrs. R. W. in your antenatal clinic (ANC); she is a twenty-eight-year-old pregnant woman in her second pregnancy. She is now at eleven weeks' gestation; her community midwife has made an appointment with ANC to discuss her dermoid cyst, which has been getting bigger as per recent scan.

Part 1

1. Take a full history.

2. How you going to evaluate the cyst further?

3. Plan her treatment.

4. Justify your plan, and discuss the pros and cons.

Part 2

1-What is the implication on the pregnancy if she decided not to have any intervention?

2-What is the possible long-term effect of complication of the cyst on future reproduction?

Examiner Instruction

This twenty-eight-year-old woman is eleven weeks' gestation with left dermoid cyst measuring 65 mm by 55 mm; the right ovary was normal, and there was no free fluid in the pouch of Douglas. At seven weeks the measurement was 35 mm by 35 mm and recently causing constant pain in the left iliac fossa, specially on walking or any activities and sometimes associated with sharp pain radiating to the left leg.

This cyst was diagnosed during last pregnancy, but the patient chose not to have any surgical intervention and preferred to have the operation after delivery. However, she got pregnant again just a few weeks prior to her scheduled operation, and it was an unplanned pregnancy.

She was planning to have sterilisation and was told that she can delay her operation until she is thirty-six weeks' gestation to have CS and tubal ligation in addition to left cyst oophorectomy.

Further investigation to exclude malignant changes were undertaken, and CA125 was normal, LDH was normal, and MRI study did not indicate any malignant features.

Marking Sheet

1-Full gynaecological and obstetric history

    Periods regularity

    Pain during period and outside the periods

    Dyspareunia

    Imaging review during last pregnancy and after   0 1 2 3 4 5

2-Plan treatment

    Laparoscopy at twelve to thirteen weeks and ovarian cystectomy

    Laparoscopy/laparotomy and ovarian cystectomy?

    Oophorectomy at sixteen to eighteen weeks   0 1 2 3

3-The cyst getting bigger and painful

    Soon treatment is justified.

    Laparoscopy as minimal surgery is feasible
early in pregnancy.   0 1 2

4-Leave alone

    Increase complications

    Torsion

Rupture

Haemorrhage

May require urgent laparotomy

Premature labour   0 1 2 3 4 5

5-When dealt with early, little or no implication on
  future fertility.   0 1 2

6-If complicated, might compromise her future fertility.   0 1 2 3

Discussion

Approximately 1 in 500 to 1 in 635 women will require nonobstetrical abdominal surgery during their pregnancies. The most common
nonobstetrical surgical emergencies complicating pregnancy are
acute appendicitis, cholecystitis, and intestinal obstruction. Other
conditions that may require operations during pregnancy include
ovarian cysts, masses or torsion, symptomatic cholelithiasis, adre-
nal tumours, splenic disorders, symptomatic hernias, complications
of inflammatory bowel diseases, and abdominal pain of unknown
aetiology. Earlier on, some argued that laparoscopy was contraindicated during pregnancy due to concerns for uterine injury and
foetal perfusion. As surgeons have gained more experience with
laparoscopy, it has become the preferred treatment for many surgical diseases in the gravid patient. A guideline from the Society of
American Gastrointestinal and Endoscopic Surgeons, published in
2011, makes the following recommendation:

Laparoscopy is safe and effective treatment in gravid patients with symptomatic ovarian cystic masses. Observation is acceptable for all other cystic lesions provided ultrasound is not concerning for malignancy and tumor markers are normal. Initial observation is warranted for most cystic lesions <6 cm in size (Low quality of evidence; Strong recommendation). Most masses in pregnancy appear to have a low risk for both malignancy and acute complications and, thus, may be considered for expectant management.

The incidence of adnexal masses during pregnancy is 2%. Most of these adnexal masses discovered during the first trimester are functional cysts that resolve spontaneously by the second trimester. 80% to 95% of adnexal masses $\leq$ 6 cm in diameter in pregnant patients spontaneously resolve; therefore nonoperative management is warranted in such cases.

Persistent masses are most commonly functional cysts or mature cystic teratomas with the incidence of malignancy reported at 2% to 6%. Historically, the concern over malignant potential and risks associated with emergency surgery have led to elective removal of masses that persist after 16 weeks and are > 6 cm in diameter. Recent literature supports the safety of close observation in these patients when ultrasound findings are not concerning for malignancy, tumor markers (CA125, LDH) are normal, and the patient is asymptomatic. In the event that surgery is indicated, various case reports support the use of laparoscopy in the management of adnexal masses in every trimester. Perhaps more informative, a retrospective review of 88 pregnant women demonstrated equivalent maternal and fetal outcomes in adnexal masses managed laparoscopically and by laparotomy.

Ten to 15% of adnexal masses undergo torsion. Laparoscopy is the preferred method of both diagnosis and treatment in the gravid patient with adnexal torsion. Multiple case reports have confirmed safety and efficacy of laparoscopy for adnexal torsion in pregnant patients. If diagnosed before tissue necrosis, adnexal torsion may be managed by simple laparoscopic detorsion. However, with late diagnosis of torsion adnexal infarction may ensue, which can result in peritonitis, spontaneous abortion, preterm delivery and death. The gangrenous adnexa should be completely resected and progesterone therapy initiated after removal of the corpus luteum, if less than 12 weeks' gestation. Laparotomy may be necessary as dictated by the patient's clinical condition and operative findings.

The surgical management of this patient is indicated due to the fact that the cyst is enlarging and became symptomatic. Laparoscopic approach is preferred at this gestation.

References

1- Society of American Gastrointestinal and Endoscopic Surgeons. Guidelines for Diagnosis, Treatment, and Use of Laparoscopy for Surgical Problems during Pregnancy.

2-Kammerer, W. S. (1979) Nonobstetric surgery during pregnancy. *The Medical Clinics of North America* 63:1157–1164.

3-Kort, B; Katz, V. L.; Watson, W. J. (1993) The effect of nonobstetric operation during pregnancy. *Surgery, Gynecology & Obstetrics* 177:371–376.

Obstetrics OSCE Station

Gestational Diabetes

Candidate Instruction

M. M. is a forty-one-year-old pregnant woman, presented to you in the antenatal clinic at sixteen weeks' gestation. She is para 2, delivered by lower segment CS (LSCS).

Her BMI is 48, and her BP 166/74 mmHg.

She has been on metformin 1 000 mg twice daily for the last few years.

1-Discuss her risk/s.

2-Plan her management during antenatal periods.

3-Plan her labour and delivery and complications.

4-Discuss the postpartum care and long-term plan.

Examiner Instructions

A forty-one-year old woman known to have type 2 diabetes, patient M. M. has two children delivered at thirty-eight weeks' gestation with CSs. She is currently on metformin 1000 mg twice daily. She was booked by the community midwife at ten weeks' gestation and has been in touch with the diabetic nurse for advice on maintaining normal glycaemia with diet and metformin. She was sent to the consultant clinic for advice on a number of issues, as she is high-risk patient. She is overweight with a BMI of 48, previous two LSCSs, and her blood sugar is fluctuating.

She is now is sixteen weeks' gestation; her BP is 160/74 mmHg. Her blood-sugar records showed variable control. She was given dietary advice and was referred to combined diabetic clinic. The plan for her pregnancy is as follows:

1- Frequent antenatal visits; watch for preeclampsia and infection.

2- Serial scans for foetal growth; watch for growth retardation and macrosomia.

3- Make her an appointment to see the dietician.

4- She is booked for an elective CS at thirty-eight to thirty-nine weeks gestation.

5- Antenatal thromboembolic prophylaxis was discussed, as she she has more than two risk factors.

6- LSCS should be performed by senior obstetrician.

7- She has been referred to consultant anaesthetist for assessment.

8- She was counselled for sterilisation.

9- Prophylactic antibiotics.

10-Watch for PPH.

Marking Sheet

Patient risks include the following:

Poor control of diabetes, retinopathy, nephropathy

Thromboembolism

Pregnancy-induced hypertension

Infections and complication   0 2 4 6 8

Plan antenatal care:

Combined diabetic clinic

Dietary advice

Frequent antenatal visits

Frequent scans for foetal growth

Anaesthetic assessment   0 1 2 3 4 5

Labour and delivery

Elective LSCS at thirty-nine weeks by senior obstetrician.

Discuss sterilisation.

Watch for PPH.

Prophylactic antibiotics.

Thromboembolic prophylaxis   0 1 2 3 4 5

Postpartum and long-term care

Contraception

Diabetic control   0 1 2

Discussion

In its chronic forms, diabetes is associated with long-term vascular complications, including retinopathy, nephropathy, neuropathy, and vascular disease. Approximately 650 000 women give birth in England and Wales each year, and 2–5 percent of pregnancies involve women with diabetes. Approximately 87.5 percent of pregnancies complicated by diabetes are estimated to be due to gestational diabetes (which may or may not resolve after pregnancy), with 7.5 percent being due to type 1 diabetes and the remaining 5 percent being due to type 2 diabetes. The prevalence of type 1 and type 2 diabetes is increasing. In particular, type 2 diabetes is increasing in certain minority ethnic groups (including people of African, black Caribbean, South Asian, Middle Eastern, and Chinese family origin).

Diabetes in pregnancy is associated with risks to the woman and to the developing foetus. Miscarriage, preeclampsia, and preterm labour are more common in women with preexisting diabetes. In addition, diabetic retinopathy can worsen rapidly during pregnancy. Stillbirth, congenital malformations, macrosomia, birth injury, perinatal mortality, and postnatal adaptation problems (such as hypoglycaemia) are more common in babies born to women with preexisting diabetes.

Good communication between health-care professionals and women is essential. It should be supported by evidence-based written information tailored to the woman's needs. Treatment and care, and the information women are given about it, should be culturally appropriate. It should also be accessible to women with additional needs, such as physical, sensory, or learning disabilities and to women who do not speak or read English.

General management of DM in pregnancy includes the following:

- If it is safely achievable, women with diabetes should aim to keep fasting blood glucose between 3.5 and 5.9 mmol/litre and one-hour postprandial blood glucose below 7.8 mmol/litre during pregnancy.

- Women with insulin-treated diabetes should be advised of the risks of hypoglycaemia and hypoglycaemia unawareness in pregnancy, particularly in the first trimester.

- During pregnancy, women who are suspected of having diabetic ketoacidosis should be admitted immediately for level 2 critical care, where they can receive both medical and obstetric care.

- Women with diabetes should be offered antenatal examination of the four-chamber view of the foetal heart and outflow tracts at eighteen to twenty weeks.

- Women with diabetes may be advised to use metformin as an adjunct or alternative to insulin in the preconception period and during pregnancy, when the likely benefits from improved glycaemic control outweigh the potential for harm. All other oral hypoglycaemic agents should be discontinued before pregnancy, and insulin substituted.

- Healthcare professionals should be aware that data from clinical trials and other sources do not suggest that the rapid-acting insulin analogues (aspart and lispro) adversely affect the pregnancy or the health of the foetus or newborn baby.

- Pregnant women with preexisting diabetes should be offered retinal assessment by digital imaging with mydriasis using tropicamide following their first antenatal clinic appointment and again at twenty-eight weeks if the first assessment is normal. If any diabetic retinopathy is present, an additional retinal assessment should be performed at sixteen to twenty weeks.

- If renal assessment has not been undertaken in the preceding twelve months in women with preexisting diabetes, it should be arranged at the first contact in pregnancy. If serum creatinine is abnormal (120 micromole/litre or more) or if total protein excretion exceeds 2 g/day, referral to a nephrologist should be considered. Thromboprophylaxis should be considered for women with proteinuria above 5 g/day (macroalbuminuria).

Pregnant women with diabetes should be offered ultrasound monitoring of foetal growth and amniotic fluid volume every four weeks from twenty-eight to thirty-six weeks. Routine monitoring of foetal well-being before thirty-eight weeks is not recommended in pregnant women with diabetes, unless there is a risk of intrauterine growth restriction. Women with diabetes and a risk of intrauterine growth restriction (macrovascular disease and/or nephropathy) will require an individualised approach to monitoring foetal growth and well-being.

Pregnant women with diabetes who have a normally grown foetus should be offered elective birth through induction of labour, or by elective CS if indicated, after thirty-eight completed weeks.

Women with diabetes and comorbidities such as obesity or autonomic neuropathy should be offered an anaesthetic assessment in the third trimester of pregnancy. If general anaesthesia is used for the birth in women with diabetes, blood glucose should be monitored regularly (every thirty minutes) from induction of general anaesthesia until after the baby is born and the woman is fully conscious.

Women with multiple risk factors for VTE, even those who are not known to have a thrombophilia or a previous VTE, may be at greatly increased risk of VTE in pregnancy. Indeed, over age 35 years, obesity and caesarean section contribute most substantially to the rates of VTE because of their high (and increasing) prevalence. Obesity warrants particular consideration as a risk factor, as highlighted by *Saving Mothers' Lives*. Twelve of the 33 women (36 percent) who died from pulmonary embolism in the UK between 2003 and 2005 were obese (BMI greater than 30). This patient has age, obesity, and diabetes as the main risk factors and warrants antenatal prophylaxis.

Babies of women with diabetes should be kept with their mothers, unless there is a clinical complication or there are abnormal clinical signs that warrant admission for intensive or special care. Blood glucose testing should be carried out routinely at two to four hours after birth in babies of women with diabetes. Blood tests for polycythaemia, hyperbilirubinaemia, hypocalcaemia, and hypomagnesaemia should be carried out for babies with clinical signs.

Babies of women with diabetes should have an echocardiogram performed if they show clinical signs associated with congenital heart disease or cardiomyopathy, including heart murmur. The timing of the examination will depend on the clinical circumstances.

Babies of women with diabetes should be admitted to the neonatal unit if they have the following:

- hypoglycaemia associated with abnormal clinical signs

- respiratory distress

- signs of cardiac decompensation due to congenital heart disease or cardiomyopathy

- signs of neonatal encephalopathy

- signs of polycythaemia and are likely to need partial exchange transfusion

- need for intravenous fluids

- need for tube feeding (unless adequate support is available on the postnatal ward)

- jaundice requiring intense phototherapy and frequent monitoring of bilirubinaemia

- born before thirty-four weeks (or between thirty-four and thirty-six weeks if dictated clinically by the initial assessment of the baby and feeding on the labour ward)

Lifestyle advice including dietary modification is the primary intervention in all women diagnosed with gestational diabetes. However, 7–20 percent of women will fail to achieve adequate glycaemic control with diet and exercise alone: oral hypoglycaemic agents or insulin will be required to control their gestational diabetes. Both glibenclamide and metformin are effective treatments for gestational diabetes. Langer et al. demonstrated that a treatment strategy starting with glibenclamide (known in the United States as glyburide) and requiring progression to insulin in around 4 percent of cases was associated with similar birth outcomes to a strategy involving initial treatment with insulin. Since then, multiple studies have shown the need for insulin

in about 20–30 percent of patients who were initially started on glibenclamide and metformin, with those requiring insulin having a higher fasting glucose. More recently, Rowan et al. demonstrated that treatment with metformin resulted in similar outcomes to initial insulin treatment in gestational diabetes, although 46 percent of women in the metformin arm required supplemental treatment with insulin owing to inadequate glycaemic control. Metformin treatment was also associated with lower maternal weight gain.

References

1- NICE Guideline. *Diabetes in Pregnancy.* NICE CG63.

2- RCOG. "Diagnosis and Treatment of Gestational Diabetes." *Scientific Impact Paper* 23. 2011.

3- Green Top Guideline. "Thrombosis and embolism during pregnancy and the puerperium: reducing the risk. *Green Top Guideline* 37a. 2004.

4- NICE Guideline, *Venous Thromboembolism.* 2008.

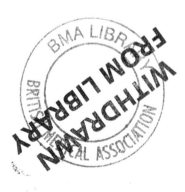

Printed in Great Britain
by Amazon